In reading Janette Moffatt reminded of our times with our neighbors over twenty years ago in East Lansing, Michigan. Jan and Bill were hardworking parents and good neighbors—Bill, an educator at Michigan State University, and Jan, wife, mother, and caring neighbor. Then a tragedy, or two, or three, or more, occurred. We know their family and watched their interactions, developments, and turmoil as a family experienced all the personal tragedy following the automobile accident that left one son, David, with a brain injury and a grim prognosis, followed four years later by the tragic death of Douglas, combined with recounting deep personal experiences in life that separated them from their belief system and faith for a time. The entire family encountered these real life happenings and learned lessons of caregiving and care receiving—lessons that can only be received and learned through an openness to trusting God's wisdom.

The Humpty Dumpty Syndrome could truly be expanded into a total life experience for Jan in her walk through life as described in this book for caregivers. She has learned the fact that "God is love and he who dwells in love dwells in God and God in him" (I John 4: 16). For without our Lord Jesus' love, the end of this story could have been the end of a family. But through Jan's rediscovery of the Holy Spirit and the working through of her life experiences and tragedies, she has become a caregiver who has learned that Jesus said, "I will never leave you or forsake you" (Hebrews 13:5). He is there all the time. The Lord will not do by a miracle what we are to do by obedience. She was obedient and worked through her personal tragedies. She learned that grace is the *love* and *mercy* of God in action. Mercy is negative, and love is positive; both together mean grace and His grace is sufficient. To show mercy by giving and caring is to love without reservation. "But the fruit of the Spirit is love," and is manifested in "joy, peace, patience, kindness, goodness, faithfulness, gentleness, and self-control" (Galatians 5: 22).

In reawakening her love and personal experiences with her entire family, Jan has discovered (as John Eldredge discovered in his book *Waking the Dead)* that from God's reservoir of love, one must walk with God, receive God's intimate counsel, take His wisdom with revelation, and accept the deep restoration that He has for each of us as we walk in the Spirit. We know that there is spiritual warfare going on for our very existence and we must be still and know that He is God. You will discover for yourself, as Jan has discovered from reliving her life's experiences in caregiving and care receiving, that the glory of God is revealed when man is fully alive, when that empty spot that has been hardened in his heart is broken and filled by the Spirit of our Lord God. We all long for something deep within our soul…within our heart's desire. When you are open to the Spirit, experience the application of the cross in your life, and put your all on the altar—as Jan has done in her walk through life and that she has shared with us—the Holy Spirit will fill that void in our heart with the love of God.

Jan's experiences and what she has learned in caregiving and care receiving are a revelation of God. Through her life's walk she overcame the many trials, rejections, hurts, and tragedies that she has encountered by walking in the Spirit. The experiences and the solutions she learned from trusting God could be beneficial to caregiver family members who are searching for solutions to yet unresolved personal difficulties and tragedies. Proverbs 3: 5–6 tells us: "Trust in the Lord with all your heart and lean not on your own understanding. Acknowledge Him in all your ways and He will set your path straight." This is what Jan has learned! This novel, representing her life up to this time, could be a sequel to *The Humpty Dumpty Syndrome.*

—FRED C. TINNING, PHD
RETIRED MEDICAL COLLEGE PRESIDENT AND PROFESSOR

A Caregiver's
TRIUMPH

JANETTE WARRINGTON

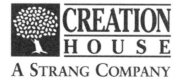

CREATION
HOUSE
A STRANG COMPANY

A CAREGIVER'S TRIUMPH by Janette Warrington
Published by Creation House
A Strang Company
600 Rinehart Road
Lake Mary, Florida 32746
www.creationhouse.com

Disclaimer: My contributors, my publisher, and I take no responsibility for any medical, spiritual, psychological or other advice offered
here.

Unless otherwise noted, all Scripture quotations are from the King
James Version of the Bible

Scripture quotations marked NIV are from the Holy Bible, New International Version. Copyright © 1973, 1978, 1984, International Bible
Society. Used by permission.

Scripture quotations marked NAS are from the New American Standard Bible. Copyright © 1960, 1962, 1963, 1968, 1971, 1972, 1973,
1975, 1977 by the Lockman Foundation. Used by permission. (www.
Lockman.org)

Scripture quotations marked RSV are from the Revised Standard
Version of the Bible. Copyright © 1946, 1952, 1971 by the Division
of Christian Education of the National Council of the Churches of
Christ in the USA. Used by permission.

Cover design by Terry Clifton

Library of Congress Control Number: 2004117408
International Standard Book Number: 1-59185-793-7

05 06 07 08 09— 987654321
Printed in the United States of America

This book is dedicated to: my parents, Wyman and Francis Moffatt; extended caregivers Rosella McComb and Marjorie Edwards; and my grandmother, Mollie Smith, all of whom are now deceased. And finally to all caregivers who give so much of themselves beyond all monetary value, including my husband and children.

Contents

Prologue

WHAT MORE NOURISHING feast could we possibly share than one that casts vision for the value of caring for another and inspires deeper commitment to protecting and enhancing the lives of others.

Some of the accounts and composites here are stirring. Others are disturbing. To protect identities, names of people and places have been changed. In some cases, the events happened fifty or sixty years ago. In other cases, the events are much more recent. Even the names of some of the contributors have been changed or not mentioned to protect their identities or the identities of others. Those mentioned in this book, fictitious or real, are not necessarily of the same faith as the author or the publisher. Any relationships or names that sound similar are coincidental and could have been drawn from a variety of unrelated material added for privacy.

Also, because some accounts of the events were written from memory, some of the details of events have been lost. However, what we may learn from these events remains so clear that they are sure to open hearts wide to the ministry of caring for others.

Preface

EACH PERSON IS just one phone call, one doctor's diagnosis, or one newborn's cry away from being instantly thrust into the role of being a caregiver. This is especially true today because modern medicine now often hands people a lifetime of being a caregiver instead of their loved ones' death certificates they would have received a few decades ago.

In today's world, few of us will escape being in the role of a caregiver. Some of us will suddenly be cast into the world of caring for a spouse disabled from injury, others will care for a parent disappearing into the degeneration of Alzheimer's, others will face the years of giving round-the-clock care to a small child struck by physical or mental handicap. In fact, some of us will be caregivers to more than one person over the course of our lifetimes.

Even those rare people who are never be called upon to be a caregiver during their lifetimes will be surrounded by other people who have heard and responded to the sound of the alarm that is calling out to them to be someone's caregiver.

As medicine continues to advance and the lifespan of the injured lengthen, we are individually and corporately challenged to respond to the caregiver and the care-receiver. Long ago, Jesus set the standard for us when He said, "I tell you the truth, whatever you did for one of the least of these brothers of mine, you did for me." Matthew 25:40

This life-story illustrates the sudden horror of the phone call every parent dreads and the lifelong loving support of God and His church that followed. It also takes you to a mental hospital where you will see that simple worship was even possible in the midst of appalling standards of care during the era of the Great Depression or when one is in the death grip of cancer.

Applying her expertise, Dr. Warrington provides both theological and psychological insight as she weaves together her life's experiences, visions, and prophecies to show the challenges that care-giving presents the church, its workers, and its members. Much is handled well in the modern church, but this book shows the room and need for new approaches. It is in all our best interests to make sure that we as churches and individuals are ready when the role of caregiver comes to us or to others.

—STEPHEN R. W. COOPER, PHD

Introduction

OUR NIGHTMARE REGARDING David began in the late hours of July 3, 1975. Screaming sirens raced to his fragile body to help. His body lay twisted between bent metal and broken glass when his car hit a tree. After intensive care, he was moved to a physical therapy hospital. Diagnosis: brain stem damage. The effects would be crippling and lifelong. The accounts of his injury and recovery are detailed in The Humpty Dumpty Syndrome.[1]

Two chapters of this book deal with David, who has lived with my husband Bill and I for over twenty-seven years. He can only be left alone for short periods of time. Hired private caregivers helped our family through some shocking and traumatic times over the years and provided an active therapy program that monitored David's free time. At times it was grueling, at other times we laughed at ourselves as we struggled together. Two chapters describe our interactions with David in a direct way, but the rest of the book reveals ways in which God prepared for me what was to come and shaped me through what did come. My hope is that the story of my journey will encourage you in yours.

The book opens with Bill, David, and me adjusting to a new caregiver en route to Huntersville, Georgia, where we lived for six months each year. We were returning from our lake home in Traverse City, Michigan, where we lived the other six months each year.

❧ 1 ❧

Realizing Something Is Amiss

THE OUTSIDE DOOR swung open. Bill stomped fresh snow off his feet. The sharp air had flushed his cheeks, adding to his anxious look.

He breathlessly stammered, "It's slippery! There are no 'maybes' about it. We must go. There's salt on the freeway. Let's head out right now. Let's go, go, go!"

I chuckled to myself. My loving husband, a willing but drafted caregiver who had been born without a sense of rhythm, had almost mimicked a rhyme from the Dr. Seuss book, *The Cat in the Hat*, I had read to my grandchildren. "It's time to go. Go, go, go, go, go!"

Bill continued, "I wish we had this trip behind us."

"I do too." Smiling, I nodded instead of reminding him that during our New Year's prayer the night before we had asked God to protect us. It was January 2, 1985; Bill had officially retired from Michigan State University just a month before. We had once dreamed of his time of retirement being just the two of us finally put the chaos in our lives behind us. But this was not to be. My adopted son David, who had been brain injured in a terrible car accident more than eight years earlier, would be making his home with us.

I heard the loud muffler of an old clunker pull up in the driveway. It the new caregiver we had hired to help us with David. We had met him a month earlier when David came home from the evaluation center for brain-injured individuals. After eight and a half years David's prognosis was that he would never fully recover from his injuries. We knew that although the house would be crowded, we would find a way

3

to make it work. David needed us. We would build an addition on to our Georgia home in a beautiful retirement community that was nestled in an orange grove where the blossoms perfumed the air and shut out any hint of pollutants from the vehicles that clogged the winter streets in the developed Huntersville area.

Now, the motor home was loaded and ready to go, and our brand-new Chevette was hitched in place to tow behind us. My husband looked out the window as Casey came into the house.

"You think your car will get you to Georgia?" Bill asked.

"Oh yes," Casey boasted. "There's no problem. The motor's in good shape. Everything is all set."

Because our traveling experiences with David had been hectic in the past, Bill was nervous about David riding separately from us in Casey's car.

As we gave the house one last check, my Aunt Marjorie, who had been a loving mentor to me during my high school years, called to say goodbye. In fact, all of our children called or stopped over to say goodbye.

I could not help but be reminded of the fact that most of David's friends had been concerned and supportive right after his accident. However, as is to be expected in these kinds of situations, they went on with their lives and began spending less and less time with him. We hoped our newly hired caregiver would be our answer—not only to relieve us, but also to be a friend who would help curtail monitor David's exaggerated behavior. We were confident the match would be a good one because Casey was so cheerful, easygoing, and likeable.

When we got on the road at last, I noticed that Bill was more nervous than I had ever seen him. I took a deep breath to try to clear my own mind of worry. We couldn't take any more accidents in our family. In 1979, our son Douglas, at 24 years old, had fallen to his death from a high tower. After David's accident in 1975 and Douglas' death just four years later, peace and balance were our only desires.

As we drove along the icy neighborhood streets to get to the highway, I couldn't help but notice how the houses were all buttoned up and quiet after the 1984 Christmas glitter. Decorations were hung over troughs, around covered stoops, and over the front entries. Backyard patios were covered with snow and hardly visible from the street.

Now that we were underway, maybe our trip would be as safe and easy as the dancing flowers in our yard in the springtime. Oh, how I hoped for this because many of our past travels with David had turned out to be anything but easy. Instead, it had usually seemed like anything that could go wrong did go wrong.

"Please God," I prayed, "let this trip go smoothly."

To diffuse my stress, I allowed my mind to wander back to the vegetable gardens my father plowed when I was a child during the depression. He had been the neighborhood fix-it man and general caregiver. During those hard times our family fared better than many others. His horse-drawn plow kept many a table from being bare of food; our cow provided milk, butter and cheese, and our chicken laid eggs for us to sell to people who would otherwise have none. My dad even provided the town with fun and entertainment by using our horse to give hayrides to the whole neighborhood each fall. I had not known then that watching my father in the role of caregiver to our community would help prepare me to be a caregiver to others later in my life.

Mothers and grandmothers watched us from their porches, where spring roses and lilacs could climb their porch rails in spring and summer. The mothers and grandfathers sitting on the porches were the hunters and watchers, scanning the outposts and secret places of the neighborhood to keep the weak from falling prey. Once a child had been raped and murdered in the woods a couple of miles away. All watchers kept their ears open for information. They closely examined the peddlers and advertisers who might be allowed into the inner sanctuary of the home. Little ones could sit at their feet and dream while trying to coax moms to purchase candy and other goods from the door-to-door peddlers. My mother always tried to buy something from them because she knew each one had a family to feed as well.

Peddlers would walk up to the porches of homes to peddle apples, dry goods, candy, toys, and other items. Even when we had no money to buy their goods, they would be invited up on the porch for a glass of lemonade.

My trip down memory lane was stopped short when Bill slammed his fist on the steering wheel and said, "Oh, the keys to the house are still in my pocket, and I was going to leave them under the mat for your nephews."

Our twin nephews were going to house-sit for us that winter while they attended a university nearby but they would have a hard time house sitting without the keys to get into the house.

Bill had made sure to have Casey and David driving ahead of us just in case Casey's car broke down. Casey was to be watching us in his rearview mirrors so he would know to pull off the road if we did. However, when Bill pulled over to the side of the road, Casey's car continued down the highway and did not turn around at the nearby freeway exit. As if to say that his worries about Casey had been confirmed, Bill shook his head.

"We've got to do something to signal Casey, but I need to go to the bathroom so bad that I can't stand it," Bill said (when Bill gets nervous the urge to urinate besets him).

Bill continued, "At this rate we're care-giving the caregiver. What are we accomplishing here?"

Was this trip going to have the usual twists and turns, resulting in my grasping for trips down memory lane to less hectic times?

Bill's muttering continued as he made his way to the bathroom at the back to the motor home. By the time he returned, Casey and David were far out of sight. The only thing to do was sit and hope they would soon notice that we weren't behind them. A half-hour passed and there was still no sign of Casey or David.

By this time Bill was so agitated that he was nearly in tears. "We can't get a mile out of Lansing and already we're in trouble. Why did we hire this boy? We should have checked him out more thoroughly."

I, too, wondered if his assessment was correct. We both hoped this unraveling would not set the tone for the whole trip.

Finally, Casey's old car rumbled alongside us and slowed to a stop. He and David were laughing their heads off. We were puzzled by their humor.

Bill exclaimed, "What are you laughing about?"

"We've been sitting at the rest stop up ahead for the last half-hour," Casey replied.

My husband's face turned red, almost purple. "What did I tell you to do?" he demanded.

Casey shrugged his shoulders. Really, it was just a simple mistake. Casey hadn't gotten Bill's instructions straight; after all, he had never caravaned with us before.

Casey's explanations did not appease Bill's skepticism. In a stormy mood, he drove our Chevette toward our house to put the keys under the doormat while the rest of us sat and waited. The boys' laughter had quickly turned solemn.

An hour later we were back on our way. All went well through Michigan and central Ohio as we put mile after mile behind us and made our way toward Cincinnati. When we stopped for lunch at a rest stop, Casey told us that he was sleepy. He had stayed up until 3 a.m. saying goodbye to his family. This was yet another red flag for Bill, and for me. A lack of maturity seemed to be indicated here once again.

We lost sight of David and Casey again on the bridge that stretched over the Ohio River and into heavy traffic. We stopped at the next rest stop in hopes that David and Casey would think to stop there to regroup with us. We had instructed them to go to the very next rest stop and wait for us if we were separated again. We waited and waited. Trying to reassure my husband I said, "I'm sure they pulled off for coffee. Perhaps we'll spot them if we go back across the river."

Bill shook his head gloomily. "That won't work. We'll only miss them. The only thing we can do is wait," he deducted.

I wondered if the boys would think to contact Bonnie, the home contact person who was to be called in the event that any problems arose while we were traveling. After waiting a full two hours we finally concluded that they must have gone on ahead without us.

We swung into our backup plan of leaving a message with Bonnie if we got separated. Thankfully, Bonnie was home and had a message for us. Apparently, Casey had readily agreed when David suggested that they stop for a cup of coffee. They made a quick stop at McDonald's in Cincinnati. David assumed that we had seen them pull off the freeway and would stop too. When we didn't show up, they headed to the motel we had predesignated as the place where we would stop that night. However, they forgot the name so they stopped at the first convenient place.

As we traveled, in the distance I could see green slopes edged with snow. I thought of an earlier time when I would have enjoyed deer hunting on those slopes. Thoughts of deer hunting, however, looped my mind back to places of fear, to other times when we couldn't find David. I was also jarred by memories of long and arduous hunts to find recreational, educational, and physical therapy programs for the brain-injured.

Now, it seemed, we were hunting again. In these moments, I was allowing fear to consume me. Many moments like these had been the result of turning my focus away from my Heavenly Father.

It was about eight in the evening when we finally arrived at the motel. Again, we waited for David and Casey. Again, there was no sign of them. We called our relatives in Michigan, but there were no messages. That night we hardly slept; we were too worried about where this new caregiver and our beloved David may be.

I wondered if there would ever be a time with more absolutes than maybes. I immediately began scolding myself for doubting that I had peace through Jesus Christ. Could it be that my doubts meant I really did not have eternal life with Christ after all?

My mind was playing tricks on me again.

I turned my attention to pondering the hopes I had for what life would be like in the coming months. I hoped Huntersville would have a church with a counselor or a pastor experienced in counseling. I felt like I had been worshipping God on the run. I believed the spiritual road on which I was traveling was leading me further away from the assurance that I was going to Heaven and further away from my God, who gives that assurance. My thirsty mind then wandered to a simpler time when I was a child and my Aunt Lillian would gather my cousins and me for times of simple worship in prayer and Bible reading. In an effort to re-create that same attitude of simple worship, I started to read the Bible that the Gideon Society had placed in the motel room. At times in the past Bill had noted that I only read the Bible in times of crisis.

Maybe he was right. I went into the motor home and picked up the soggy sandwiches and thermos of lukewarm coffee. Feast it was not! We served it to ourselves anyway.

The unknown was getting to me. I felt like I was losing my mind. Casey must learn to carefully follow our instructions. In fact, our arrangements when traveling with David simply had to be more structured in the first place.

We've got to have some kind of order to our lives.

To ease my mind I turned my attention to my hopes that I would find Christian friends who would accept, and not judge, me even though I was so overloaded and overwhelmed.

Please, God, keep the boys safe!

At last I drifted off to sleep.

❦ 2 ❧

Recognizing the Need for Deeper Connection With God

I N THOSE MOMENTS, and in others like them, I began to realize that I was in need of a much deeper connection with my Heavenly Father. Simply caring for another was not enough. Attending church services was not enough either. I needed more. I needed something that would sustain me—and my assurance in my eternal relationship with the Lord—through the hard times.

By definition, I was a caregiver. I was not the type of caregiver who responds only to a critical need at the site of a car accident until an ambulance arrives. I was also not a type of caregiver who cares for a loved one for only a few days or weeks. I was not a doctor, or a nurse, or a sitter who provided a few hours relief to families or live-in attendants. I did not work for a government entity that formulates and enforces standards of quality care. People in all of these roles had helped David and helped us over the years, but my role was that of a long-term hands-on loved one who had and would be continuing to care for David day after day and year after year. My own brute strength and determination would not be enough to sustain me, and I knew that. *But what would?*

One thing I did know for sure was that I was burned out. I also knew that I needed support from a body of believers in Christ who would accept me in my frazzled, jittery, and disillusioned state. I knew I had to be cautious in my frazzled state, however, because I suspected that if I was hit with church people's demands that I adhere to regimented church schedules, I might suffer more from the place where I was seeking solace.

I needed to hear:

> Come unto me, all ye that labour and are heavy laden, and I will give you rest. Take my yoke upon you, and learn of me; for I am meek and lowly in heart; and ye shall find rest for your souls. For my yoke is easy and my burden is light.
>
> —MATTHEW 11:28–30

In other words: come to my porch and learn of me. I will take you into my inner sanctuary of a holy, gentler, and lighter life. For my counsel is easy, unforced, like a well-tuned piano in time with my simple rhythm. For I give the fingers of your soul my music to play out life's troubles, so unload your tension on me and I will give you relief. Like many caregivers, I was so burned out that I doubted my own value. I had not been regularly praying, reading the Bible, reading books that would strengthen me, or getting the support I needed from others. Instead, I had allowed myself to be consumed by concerns for David. Often Bill and I would not talk about anything other than David until we would get away by ourselves for a while. Despite this pattern, I hoped that our winter home would bring spiritual, emotional, and physical restoration.

I did not know that it had been discovered in World War II that fatigue from battle, if caught early enough, could be largely cured within a week or so with good food, a positive atmosphere, and good reading material. It was found that safety in a caring environment and proper sleep did give relief and the soldier could usually be sent back to his platoon within seven days. Of course, the key here was that fatigue had to be caught early for the needed restoration time to only be seven days. In my case, no one had been on hand to help me identify the depths of my fatigue early on.

One of the battles I had endured for a long time was David's sarcasm. Although David would apologize when he realized that his form of humor had been too cutting and personal, he would often fall into the rut of sarcasm again. His sarcasm had worn me down.

I had also battled the stress of David often getting lost. Over time we had learned our lesson about not giving as much freedom as we had been giving him, but being in a state of constant watchfulness had also worn me out and this latest battle of worrying where he was had made matters even worse.

Bill and I were both in tears when Casey and David arrived at our Georgia home unharmed. Among their other independent missteps, they pressed on to Huntersville where they stayed in a motel not far from the house. Bill asked David why they had made an unplanned stop at the restaurant for coffee. In his characteristically humorous way, David said something like, "There was a sign in the window that said, 'Wanted: a man to wash dishes and two waitresses.'" Although furious, Bill believed Casey when he said that he had learned the hard way to not trust David's judgment. Bill and I were so thankful to have them safe with us that we decided to move on.

Our decision to forgive Casey would prove to be a good one. During the six months he was with us, he was upbeat and good for David. He proved to be dependable in providing some free time for Bill and me. During our seventeen-year winter hiatus in Huntersville, we were able to enlist companions for David from hope-filled settings. These people were phenomenal in their interest and care of David. Bill was at the command post, helping the caregivers learn to lay out plans of action.

With David reasonably settled, I was determined to get on with a deeper relationship with Christ. I also wanted to be a caregiver to needy Christians or individuals who wanted to come to Christ. But first things first, I needed to position my attention on Christ rather than the daily duties of life as a caregiver.

I was determined to remain joyful. To help me maintain joy in the midst of the temptation to give in to frustration as we made adjustments to our home in order to accommodate David, I was determined to let joy reign over frustration. For instance, we hired a plumber to hook up our washer and dryer. He was very jovial and talkative but stretched a half-day hike into a three-day journey—in eating us out of house and home, that is. By the third day, our home had turned into a full-service restaurant for this plumber because we were making him snacks and lunches just to keep him at our house long enough for him to finish the job. Thinking of delicious episodes like this reminded me of the fact that we can have joy in temptation.

With the needed new structures in place, we began to think about really settling in to the routines and adventures of our new life. We returned to mid-Michigan that spring of 1986 after buying a house on a lake in the northwest lower peninsula of Michigan. A loving daughter began a ten-year stint as David's insurance-paid caregiver. Her help and developing insight into brain injury problems was a Godsend. She was a solid leader for the local brain injury support group and a great support to us during those wondrous years. In the summers and winters we tried out many churches in our search to find a comfortable church home where we could settle.

At this point in my life I had many fears but I did not think I was prideful. I was to learn that I did have religious pride about wanting to do much for God on my own terms. Anger and remorse were my companions. In this state, my attempts to make sacrifices for God were still based on a desire for other people to notice and praise my efforts. I was too involved with David's care to have time to sacrifice much else for God. Resting in a pew was often the extent of my church involvement. I felt guilt at times when the minister spoke. I was not ready to accept more commitment.

Although we traveled quite a bit and did not attend church regularly, Bill and I received much from Spirit-filled pew partners who were dedicated to helping the hurting. Many times these quiet ministers go unnoticed by the church leaders, but we learned firsthand that their simple talents bear much fruit in the ministry of the church.

Even though the church we most often attended when we first got to Huntersville had its share of whiners and complainers who came and left the church, I was without excuse. I needed to cut into some sore spots so I could turn my attention away from impressing others and toward the Lord. Could I do it?

I thought of Christ's nail-pierced hands and feet. He suffered pains for me! Maybe at a new church, I could give Jesus a great gift because

I wanted to show my love. But that doesn't work. I could not buy my way to Heaven.

I felt so out of balance. All I seemed to do was whine about the maybes—whether heaven could be my eternal hope. With Bill retired and helping with David, why did I feel so emotionally spent all the time? As time passed, it seemed as though my days were filled with the need to go get this and go get that, move this around and put that on a shelf. I found others means of distraction from life at home that also translated into distractions from deepening my relationship with Lord. Among these was the role of being co-chairman of the retirement park activity committee.

I also had a strange desire to start journaling retirement happenings and experiences as a caregiver, past and present. Sometimes the tape recorder seemed too hot to hold. At other times it seemed to freeze to my hand as I reminisced about all the caregivers that had crossed my path over the years.

Community involvement, journaling, and reminiscing could not keep me from the overriding truth to which I should have been focusing my attention: my relationship with the Lord. Moments, hours, and days in which I could be dedicating my time and attention to even simple worship and praise of Him slipped by one after another.

I was like the geraniums that my sister-in-law grows in her garden. In the fall she stores them in the cellar under her house at a lukewarm temperature. When they emerge in the spring they look dead after so many months in such a dark place. I was lukewarm just like the geraniums. But after being placed back in fertile soil, the geraniums grow and bloom, with gentle rain enhancing their chances for survival. How I wished to be like these flowers, saved by the Grace of Salvation. The only thing that could place me in evangelical fertile soil again was the connecting power of Jesus Christ. Instead, I pictured myself as a caregiver perched on a church steeple, with my burnt-out heart lost in the balance. Everywhere I looked it appeared I was gazing down the tube of little hope for my dilemma. I did not know I needed to look up to Jesus so I could stop running away and start running towards my Heavenly Father.

❦ 3 ❧

Renewing Life in Christ

A LL TOO OFTEN, caregivers try to run indefinitely on empty. This was the case for me. In fact, I would soon find out that I was actually trying to run on lukewarm water, sinking deeper with every step. Because I felt warmth from church friends, I believed I was OK. Looking back, I wish I had spent my time reading the Bible as well as journaling events. Maybe this would have happened if I had read the book, The Spirit-Filled Man by Watson Nee[1], which I now recommend to any Christian who desires a deeper talk with God.

His insights include: "A true believer can fall into passivity...for years and still be ignorant of the danger of his/her own position. He/she can become more passive as time passes; their sphere of passivity is so great that it inflicts unspeakable pain to his mind, emotion, body, and environment."

My wake-up call began when Bill and I accepted an invitation to go to a church where, as it turned out, the pastor's sermons helped me to see that for many years I had been declaring dutiful homage to some Bible scriptures while ignoring the ones that my behavior contradicted. To straighten out my priorities, I needed to discern the Holy Spirit's truth. Only then would real inner peace be possible for me, the kind of triumph that would come from the solid assurance that I was heaven bound.

Where once I knew God intimately, now I was sorting and hunting for the same real salvation that I saw in this pastor. I felt frivolous near him because my superficial attitudes of self-importance were illuminated by his own deep faith. Through this pastor, God was coaxing and guiding me. God was calling me to hunt for His heart of hearts, to search Him for that much deeper place that would change me from the lukewarm Christian I had been for far too many years.

A pattern of lukewarmness, compromising the right for a little wrong when a lull takes place, can begin when we are children.

War Games

One example may be seen in an event that happened when I was a child that I will refer to as "war games." I am not sure how the apple war got started near the fruit market, but this is about how it went: The older kids, including my older brother and sister, were in the apple tree. I was on the ground with the younger kids. We were throwing apples, rotten or otherwise, at each other.

Then, after we had gotten bored with throwing apples, a man in a delivery truck dropped off a stack of double-packaged soda crackers several yards away from the back door of the market. Soon, one of the older kids rang out the command, "banish the crackers from the market," and before long, the strategy for stealing the crackers began to unfold. Now that throwing rotten apples at each other no longer held the same appeal and we were in a lull, the thrill of petty thievery and giving into peer pressure began to take hold.

Along with this, our commitment to not stealing was lukewarm enough to be overrun by our desire for thrills. In the end, about to be caught, we used the tactic, "When failure's at hand, run!" Many Christians, including myself, use this tactic. This is just one example of how being idle and being lukewarm opens the door to rallying behind foolish causes. Other examples may be found in bars where men and woman are lured into illicit sex, or in beer halls where the banging of huge beer mugs on wooden tables can rally drinkers into frenzied support of any political agenda being spewed out by the latest grandstander, or in parks where young people are seduced into cults.

The appetite for a flurry of emotions may be balanced by wisdom of Bible truths, but sometimes Christians do not want to put forth the effort needed to neither dig out those nuggets of truth nor fight the good fight of faith.

Many times I thought church services were boring. I wanted the minister to bring on excitement, not Spirit-filled knowledge on how to be more like Jesus Christ. My Attention Deficit Hyperactivity Disorder (ADHD) contributed to this, but that condition was no excuse for my failure over a ten-year period in Michigan or Huntersville, Georgia, to seek the tools I needed to be all I could be as a Christian.

It was the winter of 1996 and I was still lost in the lukewarmness of going through religious motions but not really embracing life in Christ. The ten-year period of a daughter being David's caregiver during the summer months was about to end. She married earlier and deserved a life of her own. If we stayed nearby she would worry about us, and the lake property upkeep was getting to be too much for us. We decided the time had come for our six months a year in Michigan to be in a home in a retirement community that was similar to our retirement home in Georgia where we had been living for the other six months each year.

During this time of transition, Bill pressed me about the handling of our estate. I was anxious; it was heart wrenching to plan for David's "special-needs trust." Yet estate planning is important for any family with an ably challenged dependent. Bill was anxious to change our will to a living trust, and I agreed. However, we could not decide who was going to administer our estate. Again, this is a must to be sure there is potential for long-term care beyond the parent caregiver. In our case, David, now forty-eight, had the potential for a lot of years ahead. We finally appointed all three of our adult children to be administrators of our estate. They were each assigned different areas of responsibility, with the authority to act on our behalf should it become necessary.

During this same period of time a trip to California to visit with my brother proved to also be unsettling for me. He was a retired naval officer, now in a wheelchair and using oxygen. It was obvious to me that his life was not going to be much longer. I cried all the way back to Michigan, for he was going to be the first of my siblings to pass on. This made me feel even more vulnerable. We were taught in a traditional church to air our feelings, and that is just what I did to anyone and everyone who would listen, mostly on the telephone. I was annoying and I didn't care. I was hurting and wanted to scream it out.

If I were to die, would I go to Heaven? After all these years, this uncertainty was still haunting me.

In 1996, soon after the trip to see my brother, we were eager to return to our retirement home in Georgia. On the way to Huntersville that October, I developed a blistering headache. It was to stay with me until the end of December. For months, I hardly had any relief, but God had a purpose.

Serve two masters

> No man can serve two masters: for either he will hate one, and love the other; or else he hold to the one and despise the other.
> —MATTHEW 6:24

Harden not your hearts

> Harden not your heart, as in the provocation, and as in the day of temptation in the wilderness.
> —PSALM 95:8

Would the wilderness within me ever be over? After consulting many doctors and undergoing a CAT scan, I found out that I did not have a brain tumor like I thought I might have had. The eye doctor thought my blurred vision might have been from hyperthyroidism, which can dry eyes and create double vision. Because lying down worsened my pain in my head, I slept some nights in a recliner. One morning at around 4 a.m., I woke up with excruciating pain. The pain medication had worn off, I was in pain, and I couldn't get back to sleep.

Finally I asked myself, *Could my problem be spiritual?* My answer to this question was soon to come. For years I had been running from one duty to another, but had failed to be attentive to the one duty that really mattered: cultivating my relationship with my Lord. Now, pain had interrupted my running from one activity to another. I was now flat on my back and God had my full attention.

MY CONVERSION

I will both lay me down in peace, and sleep; for thou, Lord, only makest me dwell in safety.

—PSALM 4:8

I called my pastor and told him I needed Christ. Later, tears burst from my eyes and ran down my cheeks onto my pillow. I sobbed with a sock in my mouth, almost choking on it, so as not to wake my husband so early in the morning. The alarm clock ticked harshly. I began to shake, rattling the headboard of the bed. Then I heard a commotion in the other room and a light flashed under the door. I sensed a dispute of anointed bodies. How did I know that? Who were they? Who was their dispute over? What was out there? Why did I close the bedroom door after I called the pastor? My soul was agonizing. In my heart of hearts I knew this would turn out okay.

The night continued. There was howling. Was it the wind during that chilly Christmas time? I had not heard it before. My mind scooped up the thought that an angel was kneeling by my bed, reaching for my hand and stroking it. I sensed I was connected to my Savior. At about 5 a.m. I tiptoed to the next room, my husband's study, and peeped cautiously through the crack of the door to the darkened living room. I wanted to yell "Have mercy!" as my heart pounded. What was out there?

"I'm hallucinating," I thought.

I forgot about the angels and turned toward my husband, but the angel I thought might be there was gone. How did I know that? I must be dreaming, I pondered. Children hallucinate over monsters, and at that moment, I sensed I was like such an innocent child. Were my cries for my soul's healing really heard and healing me? Around me now was silence. I don't know how long I stood by the door. Then, suddenly, an impression within my inner-self consumed my thoughts. "Will you be willing to win souls again for me?"

Taking no chances I said "Yes, truly yes." The power of this sincere truth spun through my head and I began to laugh with joy. My concerns over my husband's rest made me muffle my laughter into my sleeve. But tears again stained my cheeks as I was filled with spiritual power. I had entered my husband's study like a bride stealing away to my sweet Jesus. I felt heartbroken over failed efforts I did not realize were still on my mind; my pride was hurt. I had been successful at other times but I had not pleased my Lord. In those moments I learned that our success cannot buy our salvation.

Right then and there I gave my all to Jesus to do with as He willed. At long last, there was peace in my soul. As I walked through the study into the living room, the sun came over the horizon. It was a morning of excellence, a morning of victory, a morning of commitment. Then, as the light shown through the window, a voice deep within me asked if I would be willing to help churches avoid splits.

Another question came to me: "Would I be willing to help unhappy religious people be restored as I had been?"

My answer was yes. If it meant that I needed to write, then I would. I thought for a moment of the heartache of writing my first book. I remembered all of the soul-searching and anger that drove me to overcome the unbelievable odds against receiving an approving nod from a publisher. God had paved the way for me then and He would do it again.

What happened that wintry night in 1996 may be hard for some to believe, but it changed me and it changed my life. I knelt down in the middle of the living room just as the new morning light was beginning to burst through the darkness. As the light shined on me, I knew God could get me through anything. I was renewed. I would point the way for others with God's guiding hand. It was an amazing experience that I would never forget.

The merry Christmas music the church choir sung later that Sunday morning filled me with unspeakable joy. When I told Bill I had made a new commitment, he could not understand what I meant. To him, I had always been a happy Christian.

With my Heaven-bound direction sure, I had rest in the depths of my soul. The beauties of life engulfed my mind in a new way as the days ahead sung a new happiness.

❦ 4 ❧

Unmasking the Wounds of the Past

OR A SHORT time after my supernatural experience in Christ in which my relationship with Him was renewed and the focus of my life was on Him, I slept like a baby. I use this phrase "slept like baby" for two reasons: first, to emphasize the fact that I was at peace about my eternal destination; and second, to point to the fact that in many ways I was a babe in Christ. The road to moving from being a babe in Christ to being a mature believer still stretched ahead of me. Along with that, I had spent many years living my life my own way and not dealt with pains of my past or other wounds that I suffered along the way.

My head continued to ache that fall of 1996 as we prayed and paced my missed steps. My present pastor taught to not go on digging expeditions through the past but to let the past rest with Jesus. Even so, I had to journal; I knew it was important. Meanwhile, my former pastor from eleven years earlier, John, explained that in some cases of conversion or restoration there is a replay of the past and we do not know why. My head quieted down from a fierce headache. Still, I felt like I was in a dark hole or the belly of a whale. God would wake me and encompass my mind with godly impressions and give me divine emotional healing, but I could only listen for a few minutes before falling back asleep. I was not anxious. I believed I was in the psychological hospital of God. However, healing is still a process and there was more to come.

I had a new awareness of Christian mistakes, and I journaled them along with truths from God's Word, although it was hard after such a long hiatus. Like Paul of old, no one wanted to listen to my ideas. During a phone discussion, the friend told me that in my newfound grace I was obnoxious. She let me know, in no uncertain terms, that I was not her judge. It is not uncommon for new Christians to seem worse than they were before to other Christians. Like babes, they cry and demand attention. I was no exception. If I were to continue to have friends, I had to stop this. Upsetting friends was not my intent. I felt like a wolf snapping at faults my friends had been trying to overcome. One friend gave me a couple of books by a known television evangelist in which she discusses her big mouth and suggests that others also have the problem. These books gave me some insight into my "foot-in-mouth" problem.

When people didn't react the way I expected after I shared my story of redemption, I went home with my head drooping. At times even I wondered if my sobs and tears during church services were signs of relief from my repented sins or were they part of a pity party? At other times I smiled repeatedly. My husband would ask, "Why are you smiling when you come home from church?"

Our pastor preached, "Your sins are blotted out. Don't look to the past, look to the future." This brought more smiles to my face.

But at the time I still panicked, thinking that if I misstepped I would lose my salvation where God is only a prayer away to give forgiveness. I was always worrying I would get out of the Spirit. Fear of God often ruled my behavior rather than believing in His love. I would cry to Abba Father and He would help me through my times of panic.

One day my friend said, "Why do you panic and make a crisis during times of decision making?" I didn't know. I only knew that I hated maybes and uncertainties. I did not want to fail. That was it! Fear of failure had ruled me. Somehow if I failed, this told me I was not a person. Yet there was more. In some cases, I did not know I was failing or upsetting others. I would fall on my face and into Jesus' arms. I needed so much encouragement. At the time, I did not know that people with ADHD need extra encouragement because some non-hyper behavior changes require much repetition.

But was there more? ADHD has only been coined phrasing recently.

Before that it could be called laziness, not paying attention, or seeking undeserved attention.

Only taking Jesus' hand in my mind and replaying problems and past events could help resolve my pain and anger. The review of these past events included ways in which I tried not to raise mayhem in our house when I was a child of eight years. I could be teased easily as a child (I still can as an adult). The teasers of my childhood still remind me of the childhood anger (temper tantrums) I was told I expressed when I was tormented by others. To avoid teasing, I often sat with my neighbors for relief.

An errand to Beana's store was interrupted one day as I bounced along the overgrown gravel path, which was filled with bugs that I made a game of striking. I thought about the tall-tales my father told the night before on our dark porch as I went along through the high roughage.

In the next moment, I cast my eyes on a young man crouched among the weeds as though he knew I would be coming along. The man did not stand up, but grabbed my arm and pulled me down beside him. His eyes fastened upon me. I was so taken by surprise that I was nearly overcome. His speech was stuttering. I felt compelled not to be rude about his unfamiliar, perverted speech. I sat as quiet as I could and let the mosquitoes invest in me their stinger priorities, not to my liking.

The man and I exchanged glances. I must have turned pale because the man smiled. "Don't you know that I stay at Grandma Condrich's now and help Beana, her daughter, with the new store building?" At the word Beana I felt less like he would cast an unholy spell on me, like in the ghost stories the night before. "I forgive you for scaring me," I said. "Thank you," he responded. "You're not a bad man are you?" I asked. "Have you ever heard of saints?" he questioned. "I think they are Catholics," I said, remembering those who were supposed to be in our neighborhood. He laughed and tickled me. "Well, sort of," he jested. "The saints sent me to show you something special." Perhaps he saw me go to Sunday school and thought that the word saint could give him some credibility. What is it?" I said. "Come with me, it's a secret" he whispered. "It's in Beana's toilet." A toilet specialty, I thought "yuk."

How did he know I would choose that path led from our protected backyard instead of walking close to the edge of the highly traveled pavement alongside Beana's store? I thought of my mother's affectionate and joyful tone when she had often told me to take the safer path.

"Come," the man said. "Don't make me waste my time. Beana could come out at any time to use the toilet."

He pushed me from behind as we moved in tandem toward the toilet. We circled around the far side of Beana's external relief throne where I was about to be a naughty princess.

"Do what I tell you," said the molester. I was bewitched, like Snow White with the poisoned apple.

It was then that the man's mouth opened and stayed open as he shut the door behind us. By then he had a spell of panting that could launch a rocket. I got a horribly, deep, slimy kiss not on my lips, as his spit wallowed me like he was feasting upon a dripping chocolate ice cream cone, that left me whimpering in a way I couldn't understand or express. "Please don't," I begged. "Just a minute more and it will all be over, you're such a sweet girl," he stammered; unworried that his voice was gurgling. His breath that encompassed the sounds of his stuttering was like a stinky cow fluid going through a trough that leads to a manure pile. With this in mind, I could not sense why this vile slipper could find pleasure in our similar toilet expedition.

"We will finish one day up in the woods," he continued as he helped me with my underwear. Toby talked of the many flowers on the road to the woods. "Do not tell anyone about this," he warned. "If you do a monster under the toilet seat will claw its way through your bedroom window screen and get you in the night." Hot tears stung my eyes. The whole experience was so overwhelming I developed a greater fear of the dark.

I realized later Toby's speech problem occurred when he became anxious, then smoothed a little, a very little, by his cunning. In retrospect, as I remember it, the experience could only be matched by becoming a tiny toilet dung bubble going over Niagara Falls with a trail of flies. I could not talk when he opened the squeaky door carefully as though I had been pampered. I was trembling even though the day was hot and muggy. He placed fifty cents in my hand and gave me a shove. "Hurry home, little shadow," he said.

What did he mean? My older sister called me her shadow when she did not want me around. I held the fifty cents tight; I never had such a large coin in my small hand before. I snuck in the back door of my house and walked quietly up the back stairs and hid the coin. Somehow, I knew Toby would approach me again. By then I realized his panting and sweating came from excitement. At the time, I did not fully sense what excitement beyond flower picking could be in the woods that would further induce this behavior. But somehow I knew he would be back.

Do children forget when there has not been penetration? Some parents believe or hope so. This happened sixty-nine years before this writing. The famous groundbreaking psychologist Sigmund Freud and his followers believe unmasking pain can bring permanent closure. Can we overcome in Christ?

We each carry permanent records started in our brain regarding the way we experience earlier events. The way we experience the world and how we adapt to it can be internalized. This ground-breaking theory is mentioned in the book, *Born to Win,* by Muriel James and Dorothy Jongeward.[1]

Further, taking off our mask could come naturally to us if we were reared in a consistent environment where we emerge secure enough to admit our flaws, which are not always evident to others. Some rearing does not always allow for basic needs to be met. The third child of six siblings, (one deceased) I had affirmation from my parents within a safe environment. I had some understanding that I was unique.

Positive relationships with authority, such as a parent, allow for a free flow of ideas, emotions, feelings, and experiences. I had this as a small child. Some analysts can seem harsh as an authoritarian figure. Getting at the truth of our masked behavior too quickly can let us down when there is not proper follow up to help us understand proper unmasked behavior that can bring about a chance at good closure. We can feel rejected, disillusioned, and hurt when others see beyond our masks and turn us away because we do not know acceptable alternatives. I sense this was happening to me starting at age seven or eight.

These perceptions and responses of early difficulties and situations start as a child and transfer through adolescence into adulthood. This is called transference. Lack of certain nurturing is a step toward displaying underdeveloped nurturing skills that transfer into adulthood as well. Replay can unmask the unhealed original relationship. Using adult logic to replay painful experiences can bring needed closure. We can see replay helped me understand how the Toby experience was one reason why I was afraid of authority figures. It was easy to think that those in authority could and would be unreasonable or take advantage if given the opportunity, but I have learned, bit by bit, that this is not the case. A pedophile flawed my memory. Much of the emotional harm transferred into adulthood.

Once, like a child, I pestered select others for affirmation when I was unsure around them. I did not understand that I was trying to affirm the trust that was almost destroyed within me because of the pedophile. God has helped me. By nature I am persistent and will keep at an issue until it is resolved. Others may not be ready for my intensity. In church, when anger accompanies persistence one can be viewed as a church antagonist by some. I believe babes or those newly restored in Christ should not be judged quickly. Jesus does break habits by filling our cup with extra mercy and loving kindness.

To me the following is also ground breaking in a sense as it is examined and coined as a model by Muriel James and Dorothy Jongeward. The Christian may ask him/herself, "Am I satisfied with what I am discovering in Christ? What do I need to rethink? What and how to get things changed? In what context do I find answers?"

The feelings and adaptations felt as a child are affection, selfishness, playfulness, and sometimes whining and manipulating in response to what is found in three parts: the natural child, the little advisor within us, and the adapted child. This is another ground-breaking phrase in the book *Born to Win*. This also is true in the Christian experience. Our natural child is convicted of sin even before we become a Christian. The still small voice, like our own small voice that echoes truth, we hear right after we become a Christian tells us to not steal, not lie, and such. The adapted babe in Christ in the Christian life is in those who have surrendered their nature to Jesus Christ and received a new nature that is more like Christ's. Love, peace, joy, and kindness are among the attributes.

"Transference" shows up in adulthood as we transfer troublesome emotions that build up from past pain. Transference has often occurred when we overreact when sore spots are touched that stem from earlier bad experiences. As this transference is played out over and over with improper eruptions of emotions, others may not understand why we use extreme behavior to address small issues. Taking matters into our own hands, even if we are right for the moment, may not resolve issues. Our attitudes can fan the flame or extinguish it.

> Now we ask you brothers to respect those who work hard among you, who are over you in the Lord and who admonish you. Hold them in highest regard in love because of their work. Live in peace with each other.
> —1 Thessalonians 5:12–13, niv

> Let the word of Christ dwell in you richly as you teach and admonish one another with all wisdom, and as you sing psalms, hymns and spiritual songs with gratitude in your hearts to God.
> —Colossians 3:16, niv

A predator who exploited me as a child was most certainly not a hero in my eyes. However, the feelings that transferred over the years from this experience were a part of my life. It was too degrading for me to express as a child, and the feelings that lingered into adulthood caused me to feel overwhelmed when I was rejected, talked down to, or laughed at.

Caregivers can be subject to self-defeating tactics. When I was trying to find help for David I became overwhelmed. Once again, I felt like a tiny dung bubble going over Niagara Falls. I got over this by going through replay with Jesus as my Counselor and sharing with others about the experiences I have overcome.

Experts believe churches are suffering from years of mismanagement in human relations. Healing centers near or within the church itself are becoming more common where among others, marriage counseling and divorced support are offered and grieving individuals can help. This is coming at a time when many in the body of Christ come from dysfunctional backgrounds and relationships. Emotional volcano-like eruptions can be avoided. A listening ear can do wonders.

Replaying my experience of being molested as a child and understanding how transferring my mistrust of this adult to mistrusting authority figures from thereon helped me to begin to find wholeness within and began to help me to integrate into church life in a healthy way. In the past, I had seen pastors as demanding more from me than I was able to give, but now my vision of pastors and other authority figures was beginning to clear.

⤍ 5 ⤣

Examining the Roots of Early Faith

S TORYTELLING WAS MY father's expertise. This was one of the good things that survived the stock market crash in late 1929 that ushered in the Great Depression of the 1930's. Factories and stores were closed. There were no buyers or sellers for goods. Companies were dissolved, and bladders bulged from standing in line at banks before they were closed. In the aftermath, dreams were gone, balloons were flattened, bubbles were burst, and thousands of family fortunes—small and large—were ruined. Elites, officials, scholars, educators, laborers, and housewives were courteous to one another to the point of always being ready to sit and discuss a worthy topic. None dared mention personal finances, however.

It was in that 1927 to 1940 era, that the Star children were born. My parents had an immoveable determination to not just survive; but to succeed where others succumbed to despair during this period. Part of the reason for their success was in the fact that they did not have a mortgage on their home. Throughout the depression of the 1930's period, the habitual systems my parents developed earlier and diligently practiced as caregivers was the sheer force that continued to feed and clothe us, and even provided a little extra.

In putting this chapter together, I believe all who have provided input would attest to this clarity regarding my parents. From there, we siblings part company in many respects before we collectively put our memories together for this chapter. Some of us remember our parents one way while others remember other things. I am not going to try to prove or disprove any dear or painful memories that each of us has regarding our parents during the Homer City period from 1936 to 1941. The events from 1943 to 1948 are sketchy to preserve family privacy. I must speak for myself in relationship to my parents during the later dates mentioned. Others may not agree.

Each of us searched for facts, feelings, and impressions to form a composite of our memories from 1936 to 1941. We did not want to replace sincerity with fiction, which would violate the child of truth and honor within us. In altering for privacy's sake, we have not gone so far as to suggest our parents grew great apple or pear trees weighted to the ground with choice fruit or grafted in nectarines to make enormous cherries or acres of strawberries too large for our mouths, but it is safe to say that our parents provided more than just shelter. There was love, music, and nurturing along with sorrows. We were shielded with happiness until I was seven or eight years old. Although siblings' memories differ, future chapters, even though still relying on memorabilia, are more true to form.

Early life left me with strong residual feelings. Until I was healed by God, I was afraid authority figures would take advantage of my weaknesses if given the opportunity. I did feel anger over some of the happenings that life dealt me. I needed to get rid of the anger. I could not shake the fear that people would misunderstand my motives and put a bad side to my good intentions. When I was willing to take risks to accomplish a greater goal, I feared some would criticize my creativity. In some cases, this was true. I acted upon zeal rather than God's spirit. I was reprimanded by my parents and by others as I became an adult.

Still, I believe my parents were superior in principle and spirit with caring, surviving hearts. They didn't forget their duty to what Shakespeare calls "the middle humanity," and they did pity and help the less fortunate.

I can be uninhibited and casual about how I dress except for weddings, funerals, and special occasions. My sisters are more conscious about how they look. Some of my siblings remember that my parents dressed up for a night on the town. My parents were quite social. My mother and dad liked to dress up. My dad reminds me of the plumber, mentioned earlier, who lived in Huntersville, Georgia.

The plumber had a house and a yard with a lived-in look. One could find tools lying here and there in some rooms of his house. He had an airplane and would taxi out of his job-related, object- ridden yard to the field nearby and fly off to the city dressed to the nines. He would have a great time making the rounds and having dinner at a good restaurant and would then fly home. When he returned to the work world, he would leave his dress suit hanging in the closet. Although on a different scale, my parents could be casual too.

While many think of my father dressing up to the nines like the plumber, there are others, including me, who remember him under a car or fixing his tractor and lawn mower. On any ordinary day, as an adult, I would drive to Homer City, about an hour from where I lived, to have lunch with Dad. We would visit a bit, and then he would take me to a tucked away little "mom and pop" restaurant where the smells of a great hamburger hit you when you opened the door. Roast beef dinner with mashed potatoes was his favorite.

My dad, like the plumber, could talk with anyone. Never talking down, he liked to lift others up, particularly the elderly. He took time to listen to their stories. If they needed him to fix something, he let them take part in the decision and the puttering to finish up. By doing this, he would lift the elderly people's confidence by not questioning their brain-power in the way that many people do. My sister's friends would come to my dad for advice. He shared the practical side of life experiences. He told me once to have a great "blah, blah, blah" so that others will not control the conversation with unpleasant topics. I have found this technique to be true. I also found it to be a cover for my pain that would not subside at a particular moment.

This accounting of my youth will show that replay and transfer-ence can also heal others' misunderstandings and emotional wounds. It will provide examples of behaviors that early identifying markers of ADHD.

I was raised from birth by my family, the Stars; father Herman, mother Polly, Joe the oldest, followed by Jill, Jan, Audene, Diane and then Chad—these are fictional names. It was after my sister Audene died that Diane (then the new baby) was born. All the Stars' children's first three years of life were stable, including mine. I believe the stable start we received as very young children has played a large part in our being relatively stable adults. Experts confirm this finding.

I was four or five years old when my mother told me that Jesus loved me. It was my first knowledge of our Lord and Savior. I cannot remember how old I was, probably five or six, when Miss Kelly, a child evangelist, came to a holiness church nearby and asked if I wanted to give my life to the Lord Jesus Christ. That was the first time I experienced the presence of the Spirit of Jesus in me. I remember being somewhat frightened to tell mother. I do not know why. Maybe it was just the devil discouraging a little girl, even at that young age.

Mother had been a Sunday school teacher in the past and was delighted. She was careful to scrub my face and comb my hair before sending me to Sunday school. Many a time I could not wait for my mother to put ribbons in my hair and would just dash off to church without them. After arriving and seeing the other little girls with ribbons in their hair, I regretted that I had not waited. Nevertheless, I usually did the same thing all over again the following week. As an ADHD child, I was so active that I often acted on compulsion, not good judgment, and exhibited the same behaviors over and over again.

I pestered my mother to let me go here or there; my restlessness was endless. I could not sit still for long; this can be an ADHD characteristic. My older sister looked neat with her hair combed, but I liked playing with the neighbor children and making rounds in the neighborhood, visiting old and young. Often I would sit on someone's back porch, waiting to be invited in for food. This did not seem to offend anyone, however. Either way, I would not have noticed if it had been offensive to someone because I had difficulty reading body language, which can be another characteristic of ADHD.

There were pressures of all sorts in that time of the Great Depression. Lack of work and the need to earn a living were the worst. Our plate always had to be cleaned regardless of what food was served. We were told the children in Africa were starving. I hated spinach with a passion. But Jill, then about ten or eleven years old, purchased food for the meals and would tease me by getting spinach and telling me that if I did not do my share of washing the dishes, when special events occurred more spinach would be bought.

I often tried to talk to Mama about how unfair it was, but she would only answer "Maybe." However, when I would see young boys taking skinned snakes (considered a delicacy by some, like catfish in the southern states) home with their heads on a stick to secure what would soon be cooked and eaten for supper, spinach didn't seem so bad.

We had ponies named Ted and Topsy. Father used to take Ted and Topsy to plow gardens. Perhaps Dad took a share of the harvests for pay, I don't know. He leased the right-of-way on the property of a power line that went through behind our house. It was also there that my father pastured our cows and horses and provided the neighbors with rent-free garden lots. There was a sense of taking care of one another, except in private matters. I was the only one asking personal questions.

Our property was zoned so we could have farm animals for domestic use: food, drink, income, and play. Our house was small, with a living room and two bedrooms on the main floor. We outgrew our main floor kitchen and placed it in the basement. This made it possible for my older brother to have a bedroom rather than a sofa to sleep on. The kitchen in the basement had hot and cold water, a sink, and, of course, a table. We cooked with gas on a two-burner camp stove. Father got new socks by the bundle from a clearinghouse for workers. We layered our socks in winter for warmth. My mother made our dresses; store bought dresses were rare. At night I curled up on the sofa with a blanket while Jill and Diane slept in a bedroom. Jill and I fought over my wanting a light on at night while she wanted it dark.

At school, children from large families discussed what their parents could and could not afford. One girl had lard sandwiches for lunch. Others had less greasy white butter; it was considered a sandwich improvement. This made me grateful for my peach- cucumber-and-mustard sandwiches.

Depression-era people went to movies to escape reality and despair. The Lone Ranger, Joey Brown, and Tom Mix were our favorites on Saturday. We helped at home on Saturday mornings and went to the movies in the afternoon, thinking of the adventures waiting. Sometimes, however, there wasn't enough money for the movies, so Jill and

I earned our money by completing chores. One particular Saturday I hadn't done my chores and, therefore, did not have movie money. That morning Jill bathed and fed the younger siblings. My mother sat and held the little ones quietly while I decided to fix lunch for them. ADHD children cannot think before they act and have little sense of what is too great a task for them. I went ahead, pumped up the gas camping stove, and then left the gas on as I went upstairs to the main floor to get a match from my dad's pants while he slept after working his second-shift job. Because the gas had built up while I was upstairs, the fire blew with such a huge bang that it burned my nose and hair when I struck the match to light the stove.

Father immediately came running to me and combed out my singed hair. His nurturing care-giving and extra attention made it worth the fright, although it was clear it had scared Dad. He put the comb on my nose, making a game of it. He laughed and said, "That's one way to get your hair cut, isn't it, Jan?" I smiled and nodded. Then he started the stove and we fixed some soup for the smaller ones who had not been hurt by the fire.

Father tried to talk to Mother. "Polly, you must watch the stove. Polly, won't you try, my dear, to watch the older children a little closer. They're still young and we can't have them blowing up the house. Will you help us?"

She looked up, gave him a sweet smile, and started to get up. She said, "Maybe we can do it if you go back to bed." Mother and I fed the smaller children. I never heard my parents argue. My father always talked to her like she was a precious jewel.

During the Christmas season of 1936, when I was nearly five years old, my father was on strike at an automobile plant in Homer City. He and others were temporarily assigned to a tree farm just outside the city limits to cut down Christmas trees. My sister Audene, the youngest then, and I got into the habit of accompanying Mother to the farm with father's lunches.

As Christmas season drew near, a very tall, husky man was added to the tree-cutting crew. He thought my father was a union worker; when he spotted my father he approached him with an ax. "I am going to kill you," he shouted. "You caused me to lose my job, and I am going to fix you for good." My father ducked once or twice as the man swung the ax, and then my father calmly said, "I am small, I know I can't kill you, but I know I can hurt you." The man with the ax in hand stopped short and looked at my father crouching forward. Instead of swinging the ax again, he covered his face with his hands and sobbed out his story of a sick wife and too many children. My father reached into his billfold and pulled out a $5 bill (he only earned $8.00 a day from a government workers' program). Dropping the money at the man's feet, he said, "Take this, you are more desperate than I. I am not ready yet to kill for money." The man wiped his face with his shirt-sleeve, picked up the money, and said, "you're quite a man, Star."

The rest of that late fall and early winter my mother would load Audene and me into the car while our other two siblings were at school and drive us to tree-cutting camp at lunchtime, armed with sandwiches and hot soup for my father and the other workers. I can still see my mother as she was then. She wore a gray, hip-length, loosely woven sweater, black tie-up high-heeled shoes, and stockings rolled down near her ankles so as not to snag them in the weed-filled path to camp.

Father had warned us that Santa's bag would be small that year, but he also told us that we would not be forgotten. When Christmas morning came, sure enough, there were gifts for each person. Standing out among the other gifts under the popcorn-trimmed tree was a box for my mother. It was a fur coat. We called it "Mama's plush coat." That March of 1937, pregnant with another child, my mother's tears spilled on the coat at my sister Audene's gravesite after her death from scarlet fever. Mother paced, sobbing, "I want my baby girl."

My brother Joe, sister Jill, and I walked with her the near mile to a school outing. On the way home, it grew colder. In her caring way, she opened her plush coat and pulled Jill and me to her like a mother hen would draw her little chicks close to keep them warm. As we walked proudly along in our practical clothes, Mama's plush coat seemed to symbolize that if it were different times, we would be dolled up. It also seemed to say that our plight would not last forever.

I learned later that my father's Christmas-tree cutting crew took up a love collection towards my mother's coat because of her caring presence in the camp when she arrived each day at noon with food and soup in hand. From the Christian teachings of their youth, my mother and father believed in loving their neighbor. As well as warming the stomachs of the crew, she had eased their tensions and perhaps even saved my father's life.

When going to my grandparents' farm for a Christmas visit, I had an asthma attack. I never had attacks at home. Many didn't understand allergic reactions. I would choke up from hay in the barn and from the musty odor in Grandparent Stars' unheated upstairs bedrooms where we slept. One night while visiting them I had a bad attack of asthma. My dad took me downstairs and placed me on a lounge. "Her feet are cold," my grandma said. So they put blankets on me. The blankets were musty and I wheezed all the more. I thought I got asthma because my feet were cold so I never took my socks off after that. Even when it was time for a pan bath, I would pull my sock off, wash my foot a little, and then put the sock right back on. We did not understand that hay and closed-up bedrooms can grow mold and that mold caused my asthma attacks. One time, after visiting my grandparents, I could not stop wheezing and my parents took me to a doctor who confirmed I had asthma and advised us on what environments I needed to avoid.

Somehow, we always managed to go to Sunday school while staying at my grandparents' during Christmastime. That was a very special day for me because the teachers were so nice. I had a crossed eye, stuttered, couldn't read, made poor grades in school, and wheezed from asthma. I was always running and jumping with hyperactivity, was able to sing a little, and had curly hair and a sunny smile. These were my attributes. I learned late in life that some of my jumpiness could have been from my life-long "restless leg syndrome," possibly inherited from my grandmother who called this "the jiggets." I'm sure all of these attributes played a part in certain friendships, but at my grandparent Stars' house I was treated as though I were perfect.

In the spring of 1941, my mother's depression deepened. Our home became too unorganized for meaningful family events such as popping corn or making cocoa to go with homemade bread. It was hard for my mother to converse. Often I would pull at her skirt calling, "Momma, Momma." She would answer "maybe" to my questions. When Father was home, he would say, "Polly, the little ones need their diapers changed." "Oh," she would say and go do it. Five children, with one in diapers, made for a large amount of laundry. Cloth diapers were washed daily and then hung up around the basement. It seemed to me that there were always baskets of wet clothes waiting for line space to dry or dry laundry waiting to be put away.

She seemed tired all the time, often sitting and holding the young ones when they needed nurturing. Dad, in turn, would do the tasks that needed to be done. Mom cooked supper for us, but one particular evening I believe she put hot sour milk on our plates. This incident carried into adulthood and made me wonder about my mother. I learned through replay that it was cottage cheese with buttermilk. But was it really? I realize now that there were other choices on my plate. Making a game of dinner, my father put sugar on my cottage cheese. I still put sugar on mine and I can't stand the smell of buttermilk. Mother would hold Diane and Chad for hours on end. I would put my feet on one side of the rocking chair and hold on to the arms, rocking with them. My mother would smile, but if I asked a question, she answered, "Maybe."

When I was in the fourth grade, Dad sent my older brother, Joe, to our grandparents' house to finish school and help my grandfather Star. With Joe gone, I began getting up in the morning to make my own lunch. Peach sandwiches, with the bread coated thick with butter, was usually on the menu. Sometimes I would also carry an apple in my apron or jacket pocket. Jill and I helped the little ones with breakfast before we left for school. Despite our problems, we had a balanced diet. There were other children who had it worse.

One day my grandmother came and seemed to be constantly doing laundry with my older sister helping her run the washing machine. My sister stayed home from school to help her seventy-year-old grandmother sort clothes from the lines outdoors and bring the clothes indoors if it rained.

My older sister had to let her homework take second place over home responsibilities while my grandmother was there. Even so, she still got A's. School was hard for me. I had to go to school because I was behind in my studies. During this period, I came home from school one day and found no mother; I feverishly made myself scarce, running from one neighbor to another. The friendly ones fed me and then would shoo me home. The added free meal I received was a less obvious way for neighbors to help. I would run through mud puddles and get my leather shoes soaking wet. Still, I would not take off my socks.

I had a friend, Darlene. One day, during my grandmother's stay, Darlene's mother invited me to stay all night. Oh, I was so happy. My grandmother helped me wash my face and hands; she even washed my legs for me. I told her I would wash my feet, but didn't. I combed my hair and put on a clean dress. My grandmother gave me clean socks and assumed I put them on. When I got to Darlene's house, I had to take my shoes and socks off. My feet were absolutely filthy. I hadn't known my feet were different from anyone else. Darlene's feet were pink and soft; my feet were rough, chapped, and black with ground in dirt around the heels. My feet intrigued Darlene and she wanted to show me to her mother. I told her mother my feet were that way because I had asthma. Her parents didn't say a word. We went back to bed. I was relieved she accepted my answer. Now, however, I'm sure her parents pitied me.

Life for our family was like the game of uncle. One way to play the game "uncle" was to pull the other person's wrist back until they said "uncle." Scared, sometimes I said "uncle" before an opponent started. Our whole family said "uncle" during those dark days.

We did a lot of covering for the downside of our family that spring. Until better plans could be made, we girls spent the summer in mid-Michigan where our parents grew up. During the ride to my mother's parents' farmhouse, Jill talked about how much fun it was going to be with Grandma and Grandpa Jones. There was a family with nine children with whom I could play just over the hill. All lived on a two-track road about a mile from the main road that led into Hickory City, the place of my mother's high school alma mater. She had been valedictorian of her class. My older sister was to stay at Uncle George's and Aunt Lillian's home. They had a son, Cousin Ken, who was two years older than my sister.

Earlier, my mother told our extended family, including Aunt Lillian, that I was the easiest to get along with when the other kids left me alone. But if they teased me enough, I would fight for myself. I cling to this memory that helped me hold onto my self-esteem that summer. I am that way to this day. I am a very peaceable person until I get enough of something. Now I do constructive things to resolve seeming unfairness or excessive demands. My grandparents' neighbors found out about a little girl at their house that summer who played in the apple orchard and daydreamed of better places and better times. One day a neighbor visited and asked me (that little girl) to a Sunday school picnic the following Saturday. I was excited. My grandmother fixed sandwiches. I went early and waited for them to get their nine children ready. My Uncle Carey Jones, who retired from being a concert pianist, made his home at my grandparents' farm. He wouldn't take me to church because I was so active. He was divorced, which was a disgrace in that day. Although my grandmother scolded me for probing, I constantly asked him questions about his divorce. My Aunt Lillian had told me that divorce was a sin, and I wanted Uncle Carey to get saved. He didn't want to. So, the neighbors took me to Sunday school. I renewed my relationship with Jesus Christ, but my mind was on Uncle Carey's sins.

One August day my father came to the farm with two brand-new, store-bought dresses. Such a treat! We were going to the fair. I went with my older sister, Cousin Ken, and the Marsh family to a county fair. Coming back, we stopped to let my sister off at Aunt Lillian's. I was homesick for mother and did not want to go back to my maternal grandparents and my crabby Uncle Carey. So, my sister and I reversed for the remainder of our summer stay. Aunt Lillian took me up in her lap and rocked and rocked. I told her I was too big a girl to rock.

She said, "I don't mind rocking big girls like you."

"Then Ken will tease me," I replied soberly. "When we hear him coming, you can get off my lap." I spent much time during those three weeks crying on her chest as she stroked my hair.

All too soon, it was back-to-school time. I was in fifth grade, a very difficult year. We children had unrealistic thinking regarding Mother's return. We did not think about the motivating forces and the many possible consequences of a mother out of the home.

I'm not sure where my father's adrenaline to keep us afloat came from. It must have been from God. But even with love as the push, no one could do what he was doing for any length of time without suffering burnout. If Dad burned out, what then?

My dad believed he could fix it if it could be fixed. He believed a substitute mother figure in our home could benefit us children. After a time our hired mother's helper got a job in a factory so we were on our own again. Dad relied on my older sister more than I realized when I was a child.

It was decided that I would go to our own school near our family home in Homer City. I was terrified that I would run into Toby again. What could he be up to? My younger brother had been taken to our paternal grandmother's house. Obviously, she was far too old to manage a one-year-old for long. Like many caregivers, she was backed into her responsibility. My younger brother grew up in her home. Two of my dad's sisters helped with his care.

It was during times at Uncle George and Aunt Lillian's house that I really learned in-depth about Jesus Christ. They went to the holiness church about three miles away from them. There, I remembered the seeds that had been sown earlier. I immediately took to Christianity. I went to the altar one Sunday and gave my heart to God. My aunt was such a wise person. During my stays with them, she filled my head with all kinds of stories about Jesus Christ and what He could do. My head was so full of stories of Zacchaeus, David and the giant, and Sampson and Delilah that I forgot for a time all the sadness of my mother.

I was sad to go back home that fall of 1941 because I knew my mother wasn't there. A sink had been installed in the preferred upstairs kitchen along with a brand new stove and refrigerator. The beds were made. It was home.

On Sunday, December 7th, we went to Brown City to visit relatives, and there we got news of the Japanese strike on Pearl Harbor. Upon return, my father was immediately notified that he was moving to Capitol City where he would work as a tool and die maker for the duration of World War II. He needed a place for his children. When we went to my grandparents' for Christmas, it was decided I was to stay at my aunt and uncle's family home while my siblings went elsewhere. The loving support given to me by the caregiving family members who came forward could never be monitored or evaluated by the monetary measure my father provided.

So, dear Aunt Lillian became my new role model. She continued to take me on her lap and rock me while I told her how I missed mother. Aunt Lillian's love was my salvation. Because of World War II, gas was rationed, so father wasn't able to visit often. There were always lots of hugs and kisses when he did come. I always asked if my mother was home.

My aunt pounded church hymns on her piano. She could chord a little bit with her left hand, but volume was the key to her success. We could sing hymns. She couldn't stay on tune, but that didn't seem to matter. We sang church hymns anyway. Sometimes Uncle George, who was a large man, would sing too. He sang completely off key. It was certainly an out-of-key trio, but no one seemed to mind because a little girl (me) was having something of home.

The Marsh's were a farm family who did not own a car. We relied on church members to get us to and from the country holiness church. One time they got confused when riding home in separate cars and left me asleep in church. They didn't realize I was missing until they got home. My aunt walked three miles back to church to find me sobbing. She had stopped at the janitor's for a key to the church door that locked from the outside only.

All alone at the church, unable to get out, I knelt and prayed to Jesus. I knew I was in the cup of Jesus' hand and that angels were close. What a wonderful thing for a little girl to have angels as her companions.

My aunt and uncle's church members had great testimonies of what Christ could do in their lives. For example, there was Brother Lott who held his hands in the air, walked down the aisle, and told how he had prayed all night for his cow that had udder fever. Everyone knew that his cows were his livelihood and that their milk often made the difference in whether they got groceries or not. He related how in the mornings, the Lord would come, and the cow's udder would be better. He was able to milk the stricken cow. The congregation all praised the Lord together for Brother Lott's victory. What simple faith! What wonderful faith! What child-like faith! All expressed the child within them!

Sister Lott, who probably had a limited education at best, always had a number of ailments. Sister Boston was a great testifier. She was often burdened. In her burdened condition, she could somehow close her eyes tightly and go from one seat to another all the way to the back of the church. There she would find some unsaved person for whom she was burdened. She rolled herself around the person until they were so uncomfortable that they would go to the altar in the front of the church. Then everyone would gather around the altar with them and pray out loud until, all at one once, God rained blessings down upon the lost sinner. I'm not sure about my cousin's faith as a teen, but he sure had a sense of humor. He said their all-at-once praying sounded like the Chicago stockyard. My aunt did not appreciate that.

One day Sister Boston was telling Sister Lott about her husband who had prostate trouble. Sister Lott thought she had it too. Sister Boston said, "Oh no, that's a man's disease." But Sister Lott thought she had it too. She was sure she had the same symptoms. Sister Boston walked off, having given up on uneducated Sister Lott. The O'Berry family provided the music. They were all good singers. There were the daughters, Lois, Donna, and Eleanor; son, Merlin; and parents, Marguerit and Earl. That country church is still in existence though now it is on a main road. I'm told that about one-third of the O'Berry family still attends there regularly or is affiliated with it in some way. When the large O'Berry family is gone, attendance is lowered.

My own descendants have been added to the legacy and homage of simple worship at Aunt Lillian's church because my biological son's four children and two grandchildren are all simple worshippers.

Aunt Lillian and Uncle George remained true to God and faithful to me. There was such love and warmth in that home. My aunt would really go to bat for me as a caregiver and loving mother-substitute. The first thing she scolded my dad about was my crossed eye, which occurred when I got tired or mad. She took me to a general practitioner, who also tested eyes, and had him fit me for glasses. A Home City doctor had recommended an eye patch over my good eye to make my lazy eye work. I couldn't keep the patch on, especially when there was not adult supervision. It was so hard to read the blackboard. To be sure the teasing from other children would cease, I lied about what I couldn't see when I was shown the eye chart. I got glasses and my eyes straightened up. However, when my dad came to visit, my eyes were so huge through my thick glasses that he rebuked my aunt for taking me to whom he believed was an untrained "quack" doctor. He yelled at my aunt, "She's goo-goo eyed!" The next summer he took me to an eye specialist and proper glasses were purchased. All conflict was resolved without aggression. The process of conflict resolution was done with the assistance of a neutral third party, the keen eye examiner.

❦ 6 ❧

Seeing the Benefits of Having Obstacles

ECAUSE MY ATTENTION deficit disorder also included a component of hyperactivity, any number of people—especially grouchy teachers—found me to be annoying. I had a thorn in my side to be sure. A disorder, but not demon-possession as some in church may label it. This thorn in my side was a genetic disorder that could be healed divinely or with medication that was offered later in my life. At the time, there was nothing to help. A sharp tongue was often the only assistance.

> And because of the surpassing greatness of the revelations, for this reason, to keep me from exalting myself, there was given me a thorn in the flesh, a messenger of Satan to buffet me – to keep me from exalting myself! Concerning this I entreated the Lord three times that it might depart from me. And He said unto me, "My grace is sufficient for you, for power is perfected in weakness." Most gladly, therefore, I will rather boast about my weaknesses, that the power of Christ may dwell in me.
>
> —2 CORINTHIANS 12:7–9, NAS

ADHD kids may act quickly on an idea that comes to mind, without first considering that they were in the middle of doing something else that should be finished first. They are excessive, loud talkers, often monopolizing conversations. For this and other reasons, when I was not yet sixteen, I decided to quit school. The following retraces some of the reasons.

One of the wisest and saddest observations I have ever heard was

47

made from a five-year old, Mary. She had been living in the country. From the time she was two, a friend from the city had come to spend his summers with her. When Mary came to the city she found herself in a nursery school group with her summer playmate. One day her mother commented on the fact that Mary never spoke of her old friend, and never invited him to her house.

> "Oh," said the child, "we are not friends any more … He doesn't like me."
> "But that can't be possible. You and he have been such good friends all those summers in the country."
> "Oh well," said Mary, "that was in the country. There were just two of us. When there are two, it's easy to be friends. But as soon as there are more than two, it is very difficult."[1]
> —TERRY SPITALNY, CHILD STUDY

This could describe me coming from Aunt Lillian and Uncle George's farm home. I had left their nurturing arms for the second time in 1944. My father returned to Homer City and wanted some Stars with him. Earlier, I had earned failing grades in a country junior high school a mile or so from our Homer City home. Now, an ever larger, city accredited school was the answer for high school. In 1947 there were two thousand kids whose social skills and self-confidence had been honed in the hard knocks of life in the large inner-city. They had left me far behind. There was very little extra help, and no one understood the problems of ADHD children. ADHD children were thought to be retarded or uncaring because we lacked organizational skills. Indeed, they believed there was a problem that discipline alone could not handle. My protocol skills were limited, and it seemed I was always in the wrong place at the wrong time—another symptom. I was considered stupid by the aggressive, street-wise children, and I often left school early so as not to be harassed. Therefore, I didn't receive the homework assignments and my grades fell. My teacher insisted I manipulated and faked not understanding assignments.

One day at home I picked up one of my dad's magazines with exciting stories in it. As I read I realized that little words made up bigger words. All of a sudden I was decoding words. I read constantly after that. My dad glanced at what I was reading, but said nothing. I'm sure he was glad to get me to read anything.

While in the tenth grade, I got caught skipping class. The counselor told me to bring my dad to school. They needed to get to the heart of the problem. I was scared out of my mind. The Dean of Women had already accused me of everything from sleeping with boys to participating in sneaking dad's car for joy riding with the opposite sex. I didn't know such exciting adventures were possible.

My father corrected the school counselor when she told him I was failing all my classes; I was not failing gym—a small victory because my dad defended me. He reminded her of my reading difficulties and that I was now reading magazines at home. She was caught off-guard. She looked up my records, but didn't apologize for her error. Then my father went to bat for me. He asked about the teacher who called me a nuisance in sewing class. I believe I talked back to the counselor and told her that there were girls who were worse off than me and they were passing their classes.

The counselor was not impressed and defended the teacher who called me a nuisance and gave me a bad grade for finishing my sewing at home where it was quiet. She called it "excuses" when I told her how overwhelmed I was in the classroom with all the machines running. My dad, on the other hand, defended me. I felt very loved and nurtured when he told her that no child should be considered a nuisance. Many years later I would learn that the troubled person is often the best source of accurate information about his/her own struggles. The answer often is not what seems most obvious. I was trying to say that my struggles worsened in less structured or noisy situations like sewing class, but she was not hearing me.

I did enjoy my American Literature class in high school, though. I liked studying the simple written words used by nineteenth century authors as well as reading their ideas about characters. Charles Reade is one of my favorites. The summer I spent with my maternal grandparents attuned my ear to descriptive vocabulary contained in his work. My maternal grandfather had been a teacher and his expressive use of words, along with Reade's, is still in my memory.

"Two men went to church to pray. One was a so-called leading citizen and the other a school teacher. The prominent citizen stood, and with eyes turned upward, said: "Oh, Lord, I thank Thee that I am not like these professional men, even as this poor teacher. I pay half the teacher's salary; it is my money that built this church; I subscribe literally to foreign missions, and to all the work of the church. It was my money that advanceth Thy cause."

The school teacher's prayer was quite different. He simply bowed himself in humility and said: "O God, be very merciful to me. I was that man's teacher."

Over the years my father's unwavering care-giving would teach me that there are times in families when we have to abide, tread water, or make the best of what's available, surrendering to the less than ideal. Much later, Bill and I also had to draw on the less than ideal when we painfully came to terms with the fact that David was not going to fully recover. By abiding with me, my father had also modeled the abiding love of my Heavenly Father and showed me a years-long example of abiding in love for others—including David.

> Happiness is a habit – cultivate it.
> —Eleanor Hubbard

> The happiness of man consists of life, and life is in the labor.
> —Tolstoy, *What Is to Be Done?*

For many years, my father had been my "parents." He had been my primary caregiver. Like my Heavenly Caregiver, my dad would patch up or overlook my mistakes. In uncovering the pain of my past, I was beginning to see a roadmap for accepting and forgiving myself, and for accepting and forgiving others.

Although he did not know it then, my father had been caregiver to someone who was ably challenged with ADHD—me. In turn, being ably challenged and receiving special care and attention from him and from other loving people helped to prepare me for decades of being a caregiver to David. It also gave me insights into how to help other caregivers understand and be more sensitive to the unique needs of those in their care.

As I was taking the Lord's hand down memory lane, I was seeing how the Lord had used this Star family member's perseverance to succeed regardless of difficulties as an ably challenged person. This prepared me to serve others as a necessary part of my inner healing. It would enable me to move forward in my relationship with the Lord, in my relationships with others, and in Christian service.

As I thought about other ways in which my father had been a good caregiver to me, I remembered incidents when he was gracious and in so doing exhibited the grace of God to me at an early age. One of those incidents was may or may not have been ADHD related. An illustration of this occurred when I was thirteen years old and I had mistakenly fried potatoes in axle grease. My father left a container that looked like regular grease in the kitchen, and my parents always coached us to belong to the "clean plate club." A younger sibling shoved the terrible tasting potatoes into the hole that had formed in the wicker bottom of her chair. My older sibling, catching on, put her potatoes in my younger sibling's apron pocket.

I was put-out because I didn't sense the deception right away, and ate a bit longer then the others. I began to cry, stopped eating, and left the table. My father had mercy on me and ended the outdated clean plate club, just like God had mercy and sent Christ to end the law for sin restoration that opened the Day of Grace. Receiving grace from my father would help me to later accept the grace of my heavenly Father, who was walking me, by His grace, through the healing process that would help me to extend grace more often to others—partly through forgiving others for things that occurred in my past.

My dad exhibited forms of grace as well, including helping me to clean up my messes. An example of this happened when I was a teenager living in One Saturday afternoon in Homer City my friend Darlene and I decided to have a small party for our boyfriends. A freshly papered kitchen would help make our home more presentable.

We followed the directions on how to make paste but there wasn't room to lay the paper out to apply the paste except the stove. We laid the paper across the top of the stove, forgetting the pilot light was on. Sure enough, as we moved the paper across the top of the stove, several brown spots appeared where a hole was about to come into existence. We did not want to run out of paper so we applied those paper strips to the wall anyway.

Out of the extra, we cut squares and patched them over the burn spots causing a few wrinkles that we couldn't smooth out. Another problem was a leaky roof that left brown spots in the paper on the kitchen ceiling. We'll paint over the brown spots, we figured. But what could we use for a paintbrush. A scrub brush would do! In the basement we found some old paint that, when opened, had chunks of crust in it. We didn't realize that aging paint could cause a problem; we thought it was the nature of the beast. We got a stick and mixed the thick, crusty paint and were ready to apply it to the ceiling. Only a miracle from God could have prevented what was about to happen. Standing on a ladder from the garage, I dipped the scrub brush into the lumpy paint and applied it to the old paper on the ceiling. It peeled off from being wet then dry so many times. The remaining paper began to crumble from the bristles of the scrub brush. We painted the plaster then used more paste to hold the edges of the paper that didn't crumble down.

While applying the paint, we paid no attention to the splattering that was dripping down the cupboards and onto the just washed dishes. The only thing to do was to paint the cupboards to cover the splatter. The paint, complete with globs of crusty chunks and crumbled wallpaper, clung to the cupboards. After evaluating the effect, it was clear the cupboards would need a second coat but there was not enough time. The boys would soon arrive. We hurried and placed the remaining paper on the walls any which way we could just to have them covered. Each application of our efforts required a layer of newspaper on the floor to keep drippings from touching the dining room. By the time we finished, there was no time to clean up the mess; we had to get ourselves cleaned up! With a splash of water and turpentine, a rushed change of clothes, and a quick run through our paint-spattered hair with a turpentine soaked comb, we were ready to greet our boyfriends. We kept the kitchen door shut during our party. The boys would not see our hopeless attempt at improving the kitchen.

We desperately hoped the dime store perfume we doused ourselves with covered the smell of turpentine. Dime store perfume itself was a powerful scent that could cover even the most foul of smells, but just in case, I consulted my sister. She took a whiff, held her head as if she was about to keel over, then assured me it would do the job. An executive had soiled his hands on a machine with which he was not familiar. Although he had a handkerchief, he thoughtlessly wiped his hands on a worker's apron, which was hanging on the end of the machine. After he had gone, the worker exploded: "Who does he think I am, his slave? My apron is as good as his handkerchief! Maybe I just work here, but he doesn't need to rub it in."

After wallpapering the kitchen, my friend Darlene and I learned something of potty training. We tried to spruce up the house by wallpapering the kitchen before a tiny party. We fed our boyfriends each a pickled baloney sandwich and licorice drink. The licorice drink was supposed to be pretend liquor. Our boyfriends soon tired of the party. We could not understand their boredom; we banged the swinging kitchen door enough getting the food. When our boyfriends took us to a movie after the tiny party, there was ice outside and the soles of my shoes were slippery. Just before we got to the theater, I slipped and fell putting a huge hole in my rayon stockings, injuring my knee and tearing my skirt. I tied my headscarf around my bloody knee and limped along behind. My seams in my stockings were straight though—definitely a plus. He also entered the theater by a different door than I. He sat near me during the movie—another plus. But to me he seemed a little snooty and when I mentioned it, he left the movie early. I lagged behind Darlene and her boyfriend as I limped along with my wounds feeling like a bandaged flute player left over from a revolutionary war of sorts—a negative going home.

I sure hoped my father, who was due home, didn't arrive early from his second shift job and see our kitchen papering before we had a chance to make improvements. When he arrived, I shooed Darlene's boyfriend on his way. Then Darlene and I ran up the stairs hoping my Dad would go straight to bed and not see the kitchen. We reasoned we'd get up early and clean. No such luck. Around 7 a.m. there was a knock on the bedroom door. It was my dad. "Go downstairs and clean up that mess," was his command. "What on earth did you think you were doing?" He scolded as Darlene and I followed him downstairs.

Darlene dressed on her way down, grabbed her coat off the hook nearby, and scooted out the front door for home. To say the least, my dad and I spent the entire day scrubbing. Dad scraped the excess crunchies off the cupboards and applied a second coat that gave some relief to the look, but a professional job it was not.

❦ 7 ❧

Letting Go of Anger, Fear, and Disappointment

UNTIL I WAS sixty-eight years old, I didn't realize how fear of authority figures was carved deep into my being by yet another terrifying incident that had happened in the middle of the night when I was a young teen thinking about my mother's beautiful singing voice. Sometimes when there are difficult incidents to deal with, pulling them into a more natural setting makes it easier for all concerned. This is my hope while remembering my mother's wonderful gift to me and her singing that blessed our family for many years.

Suddenly, around midnight while I was still half-asleep, I became aware that someone was trying to steal my precious gift. Then I heard an indistinct voice, followed by strange muffled sounds of a struggle. Squeaky noises hung in the air. Was it a ping I heard next or a gurgling? In the partial moonlight beaming in through a small window, I could see a figure that seemed to be standing guard in my bedroom. Who was it? It was moving and rotating in the shadows, but then it stopped suddenly. I was afraid it would swoop down and grab my gift like a hawk.

There was another whirl of sounds. Out of sheer fear, I squeezed my eyes shut instead of opening my mouth and crying out. Then a crazy thought hit me: *My dad would be pleased that I kept my mouth shut for once. Why am I thinking of this when I am about to lose my precious gift?* I heard something else followed by deadly silence. Finally, I heard my bedroom door close. I opened my eyes and the shadows were gone.

The following nights I listened for the sounds of footsteps and pondered what I thought might have happened. I did not tell anyone except God about the terrible scare I had that night. I sobbed and sobbed for my mother. I cherished her gift all the more, but buried the incident in time and put the memories to sleep.

Over the years this incident regarding misplaced anger seemed to be the straw that broke the camel's back. I had pushed the memories under the surface of my consciousness. The time had come for me release the anger, but only God knew how to make that possible. He guided me through this release of anger by helping my mind to navigate through the obvious possibilities until I was able to sort out what had happened that night.

I remembered our neighbor, Cora, who was in her fifties when she lived in an upstairs apartment that was right next to ours. Also, I remember her brother who visited often and was a heavy drinker. As I thought about him, I realized that when in a drunken stupor, he would have been entirely capable of coming through an attached, closed-up closet into my bedroom. The closet door had a second door in the back which, if unlocked, could access my room.

In addition to locking the door, the builder had placed a barrier there that inhibited access from one apartment to another—access from Cora's bedroom right into my room, in fact. But had he?

Then, I remembered my dad nailing the barrier in place, upset that the builder had not completed the job of removing the door altogether and boarding it up. Of course! When Cora's drunken brother came bumping along the low ceiling closet and turned the knob of the squeaky door that led from the closet to my bedroom, my dad had heard him and was expecting him. When my dad came up the stairs and opened the door to my bedroom, the drunk had slipped back into the closet.

Now, as an adult woman in 1997, I yearned to be a more mature Christian by getting rid of more emotional baggage left over from my youth. Led by the Spirit of God rather than my anger and fears that were embedded in childhood memories, I asked God to heal the long misplaced anger that had lodged in me when the following painful incident occurred.

I also asked Him to help with my feeling of bondage that had rendered me helplessness. God spoke to me, "Where's the fruit in the feeling of helplessness? Where is the evidence of lives impacted in a positive way as a result of focusing on your gifts rather than your unresolved baggage? Look around and see what lives have been changed, who has been helped and encouraged and how your church can benefit from your gifts."

Dealing with my fear of authority figures and overcoming my feelings of helplessness meant that I would need to retrace my experiences with the child molester, Toby, even further.

When I was eight, Toby had threatened to tell my parents about the incidents. Because the family was struggling so, I believed I was doing my part by not adding to their troubles. Also, in some skewed way, I thought the money Toby gave me was a way to help them.

As a nine-year-old in 1941, I faced a late summer that I had been dreading after that first incident in the toilet when I was eight. Both time periods were nightmares of Toby-harassing. I was continuously afraid of the toilet monster on the safer path to the store so I opted to walk down the shoulder of the cement highway, which, besides being scary, my mother frowned upon. What was I to do? One day after school while passing by an opening in the partially built store, Toby reached out and pulled me through the opening. I was leery as I lay on the gravel. His hot, bare stomach was point blank in my face as he crouched over me. There was no hope of recovery from the fly buzzing incident. But there was time to unleash more panting from Toby and a gangrene-like sweat from his pulsating belly button where my smeller was detained for a moment. I thought his hot, wet kisses on my face and lips must have been a symptom of dung fever. It was not celestial constancy of pleasure. Would this ever end? Toby then sat me up, brushed me off, and sent me on my way. We will pick flowers in the woods later when there is more time he cooed with a wave. "It had better be flower picking," I thought. "And he had better know the good places like he promised."

The pennies from my dad were enough for now. They bought little, but it was enough for a little girl. Even Christmas was little compared to that of others, yet it was enough. God's grace is enough. I always felt nurtured by my dad while I was growing up. Although sparse at times, it was sufficient as God's grace is sufficient. Toby described the boxes of gifts, measuring with his arms outstretched. His unholy intents were exciting in their counterfeit simplicity but his panting was disturbing and revealing. "You're thinking, again, that I might be naughty, but it's not naughty in the woods," he cooed to me. "We will play and open presents." I agreed, but his stuttering started up again and I could not understand his directions. I ran home.

There were three streets with sidewalks that led to the woods. It was planned as a subdivision, but the Depression halted its completion. The woods lots were sites for the more expensive homes. There were holes dug for a couple of basements. The woods went beyond the construction holes. The woods went so deep one had to watch where they were going or they would not see the open holes in the ground. Toby said he would protect me. He knew where the construction holes were. I could not get his directions straight. He wanted me to go down several blocks of pavement to a dirt road that led to the road where he would be waiting to guide me to the back of the woods. *Why so far into the woods?* I wondered. We did have to get past the failed construction site but there was no one around. On that route, there was a white house. I sometimes would go there to talk to a pretend friend.

The appointed day arrived to go to the woods. As I walked, I was thinking there would be mosquitoes. Toby could not protect me from them. As I approached the corner where I was to meet Toby, instead of turning into the woods, I went the opposite way toward Miss Jones' house and ended up at home.

But I did not go the round about way. Instead I went straight to the intriguing white house with a guest-chamber upstairs where my imaginary friend sat in the window. For many years, I thought she was real. But in replaying this account with my older sister, Jill, she said a little girl her age had died there when she was in kindergarten or first grade. Jill went to visit. Perhaps I wanted to go also and then later imagined she was still there. Anyway, that day she was there so I stopped and threw stones at her window and she laughed. She appeared to me like a baby. I walked around up and down the drive for a while, dragging my foot through mud puddles left by an early morning rain. As I walked,

I was thinking there would be mosquitoes. Toby could not protect me from them. In replay I approached the corner where I was to meet Toby, I smelled the fragrance of my mother. It was a welcome contrast to the malignant, oily, alienating chicken feather smell I remembered from the disturbed man. I saw Mrs. Jones' house where Billy lived, the boy who took music lessons from my mother. It seemed to me my mother was standing by their house, a short walk away. She was smiling and motioning me to follow her. I particularly noticed her smile had a halo look to it. I did not turn in the dreadful possibilities in the woods, but turned and followed "my mother". When I got home she was sitting, holding the baby. I though it was odd that she could get there so fast. I kissed her and baby Chad. Was my mother really on the road that day or was it my guardian angel coming to rescue me? I don't know what dangers faced me that day. I believe the warmth I felt from my mother's presence was from the angel of the Lord. Surely God was watching over all of us. The Bible tells us that angels watch over us.

God provides guardian angels.– Glory to the Lamb!

The Scriptures bear out that angels will even fight for us and return to complete the work when we're out of danger. Luke 10:19 states we have authority over evil. God gives us power to back up our authority. That should give us confidence in our authority given by God. Philip asked Jesus to show him his Father. Jesus responded by saying, "If you see me, you see my Father." God planned the creation. Jesus speaks of it and the Holy Spirit helps us understand it. Christ said to Thomas, "Blessed is he that believes without seeing." Attitudes of trust and faith are invisible.

Hebrews 12:32 tells us that we will come to Mt. Zion to worship with 10,000 angels. Second Peter 3:12 says the day of God is speeding His coming. An angel of the Spirit of the Lord was surely present that day.

I am not surprised God used His angels to follow me down that fateful road toward the child molester. I grieved the loss of my mother ever since that terribly traumatic day in May 1941, when I came home from school and she was not there. As I remember, it was around 3:30 p.m. I noticed my father's car was in the driveway. He had not gone to his second shift job.

Our house had seemed to hang in space. I knew something was wrong as I walked up to the back door, which was covered with a quilt. One could easily reach around a loose spot and open the locked door from the inside.

My father called me up the short flight of stairs to the living room. He said my mother had been taken to a hospital and that my grandmother was going to stay with us until school was out and then I would go to my grandparents' home for the summer.

I know my way of telling about my mother's final days with us, as I saw them, and how they affected me and mine can give a picture of the happenings but it is not the whole story and never can be. Others can tell it.

I will tell how I learned her warm, sweet ways. I remember I would have given anything to know the words and ways that made my father so happy when they were married. My mother won the respect and admiration of all who knew her. Perhaps, in heaven where the pain is all washed away, I can sit down with my mother and learn who she really is.

The day she left, I thought it was my fault she went away. Maybe if I cleaned the house, washed my dress, or combed my hair better, my mother wouldn't have gone away. I cannot begin to express the hollow feeling I had in stomach. Her presence at home shielded me from pain inside and outside in the world about me while my dad was at work. My mother gave me a sense of nurturing and safety that was there no more.

I have asked myself so many times: How could this have happened? As an adult, I learned that my father first took my mother to a ward at a regular hospital. At this hospital women were on one side of the hall and men on the other. She was admitted for depression. The doctors believed she would improve if she spent a few weeks in a sunny room with no responsibilities. They believed she would be home soon, refreshed and ready to greet friends, neighbors and family, but soon after she arrived there a very sick male mental patient, who got loose, hit her on the head with some sort of instrument rendering her unconscious. My father was not told. They took her off to a mental asylum.

Now on top of being depressed, my mother was head-injured. Shock treatment was commonly used to treat depression. I now hope that she did not have a swollen brain from her blow to the head. That takes a while to subside after injury. If she had shock treatment before her injury healed, it could have worsened the swelling. Did they know about this in the late 1930's? I wonder. There was so much I didn't know then. But swelling from brain injury does cause serious problems.

As I understand it, Dad did not know about my mother's injury until he went to see her and she was not there. He had to go to state agencies to find out where she was and then he learned that, without his authorization, they had transferred her to the state mental hospital about an hour's drive from us. It was there he found her in some kind of bleak hospital uniform. All the patients dressed alike. He asked where her dresses were that she had been wearing at the rest and recuperation hospital. They did not know. Bewildered, he wondered why she could not wear her own clothes. He found out more details of what had happened after an interment period.

One Sunday in the early winter of 1941, my father, along with a sibling and me, went to see her. A guard opened a locked gate and after parking our car we entered the receiving room. The doors locked behind us. There were elevators and still more doors to unlock before I could see my sweet mother. I couldn't imagine what was in the hospital that would require locks, but when I stepped off the elevator, I saw all kinds of people with severe mental problems. Many were talking and chattering to themselves. Some were flinging their arms about. Some were even screaming. It was awful! There were patients restrained in beds and chairs. I could not understand the need. It frightened me. My dad told me they were ill and doctors were trying to make them better.

Looking back, I remember being amazed when some of the residents went to the bathroom on the floor. And it was there that my mother, a refined lady who had been a Latin and piano teacher, was housed. In that first visit it appeared that help was sparse and mother was not conscious of her surroundings, particularly where the bathrooms might be. Did she go on the floor also if an attendant did not understand her need? My dad rang the buzzer for help but finally gave up. We then took my mother to a bathroom and washroom combined.

Later, an attendant lifted her striped garment made out of mattress ticking she wore that day and rinsed her with a hose. Then she dried her with a towel. I used the bathroom and they did not rinse me off, so I knew this method was reserved for patients. It appeared to me the patients were not wearing underwear for the convenience of the caregivers. To me, it did nothing for their dignity or a little girl who had never seen her mother's "privates." It was hard not to be embittered. It was so degrading. I could not understand.

My father waited for us to return from the bathroom and took us to the dayroom. Nine years old that visitor's day in September of 1941, I was filled with mixed emotions. I loved my mother with all my heart but I was confused. Sick people were usually in hospital beds not flinging their arms about. My dad saw my anguish and gathered me to him. He put my head under his arm coaxing me to respond to my mom: "At home, you sang with your mother. She loves you." It seemed to me that Sunday my dad was trying to make a family worship. We were so encouraged. My mother played and we sang "Jesus Loves Us." After clutching my dad earlier, the other dear family child first, then we moved on each side of mama as she nodded and smiled. In that dayroom other mentally ill individuals did crafts, played games, and visited with their families. I wanted us to be alone with her. My heart yearned to softly lay my head on my mother's shoulder and have her look at me as she once did. I wanted her consolation, for her to look at me with tender concern toward my scraped knees when I fell on the steps. I wanted her to look at my hurts as she once did, but I did not show her my pain.

We went to see my mother again just before World War II broke out. Days were short. Dark drops of rain, sleet, and snow were falling to dampen our spirits. The halls in the asylum seemed dismal then. My mother had been my father's lover and friend and my mother for too short a time.

This day my mother greeted us as we stepped off the elevator. The nurses at the registration desk must have called the nurse on her floor about our visit in time for her to prepare. She was keenly aware and smiling. My father told her it was good to see her so cheerful. When we went into the dayroom, on one of the tables was a vase with a single lovely rose. When we sat with her, she smiled with her eyes on the flower as though we were company and she was the host. She made a wonderful host when my parents had friends in our home. Her delicate cheeks were flushed and her smiling eyes melted away any doubt that I should be scared. That day she was again my mother.

As our small family gathered together, my mother played the piano. Then a woman came and stood near us. She shook her fist and said something like, "Always love me and never, never disobey in small things or great." She spoke right into my face and it frightened me for a moment. I thought I had done something wrong. My dad took her by the shoulder and moved her to another table and sat her down. She did not try to move. Then my father tenderly beamed at my mother as he put his hands on her and whispered, "Come Polly, play a song." He showed neither remorse for her present condition nor did he make excuses. My father encouraged me to sit beside my mother at the piano, but I didn't move from his side as she began to play, "Little Sunshine, Little Sunshine, I'll be a sunshine for Him." That's all I remember of that moment. Then, as before, other patients noisily came into the room with their families.

Mother's hair was not curled but still my father told her how beautiful she was and admired the rose. Perhaps she asked a nurse for it, I don't know. Was the rose really there? Or do I want it to be there? It does not matter, we were a family. Sensing I needed an extra parental touch, daddy pulled me closer. He said, "Don't let any of this bother you; we have a little more time here together with mama. You stand on the side of your mother." The other loving sibling moved to the opposite side of her. Then dad said, "I will stand in back of her so she doesn't fall off the bench." We all laughed, including my mother. Of course she was able to sit up without falling. She played beautifully: "Beautiful Island Somewhere in Heaven," and "There is a Church in the Wooded Wild." We sang out while my father seemed to mentally note every action. It was as though he wanted to etch it in a painting that could hang in his mind forever if need be. I prayed, "Now I lay me down to sleep" and my mother smiled and nodded her approval.

My father put his arms around her chest and held her as she played. She left the piano and they embraced. We had triumphed over something that day. Perhaps it was clear, we were still a family. As we were leaving we recited the Pledge of Allegiance and I said the Lord's Prayers, just as I did at school every day. We could recite them perfectly and not stumble as we did with the words to some songs. Tears welled in all our eyes when it was time to go. We must have stood at the elevator for five minutes waiting for the door to be released. We gently kissed and hugged our mother goodbye. We had enjoyed ourselves in our unforgettably simple worship together. Thousands worship in glorious services honoring Christ but none can surpass what I experienced that day in simplicity of family worship with my mother. When we rode home with my dad that day, it was like a benediction in a sacred realm without measure. I did not realize it then, but we would be moving away from Homer City.

The way in which I cherished her sweetness had been the way in which God protected me from Toby when I was on the road to being raped and losing my very life. Being truly thankful to God for His protectiond during those critical moments was a key to my becoming free of anger over what had happened and trusting authority figures. Even though I had not felt free to tell my parents what had happened to me with Toby or discuss other pains, God had been a good Caregiver to me by using my earthly caregivers—my natural parents—to protect me. It would be a long time before I would come to grips with the fact that we do not get over things by keeping them in the dark and that getting issues out into the open beats Satan.

Later, giving God my deep disappointment and confusion about what had happened to my mother were both very important steps that were preparing me to retrace and mourn some events for true emotional healing.

❦ 8 ❦

Assessing God's Call and Anointing

I DISCONTINUED MAKING MY home in Homer City in 1948 and moved with a sibling to a small town near Aunt Lillian's and finished high school. I met a wonderful farm boy with some means to provide. The whole family liked him.

After high school, I became Mrs. Robert Cooper. We had a son, Stephen, in 1954. Stephen is a wonderful person, and his wife Bonnie is a dear. He and his family are all born-again Christians. (When Bill and I married, we adopted each other's children so I have four, one deceased, other wonderful children.)

Moving along in my journey to be whole again, the Lord brought to my mind a critical day years earlier when life with my husband Bob had taken a sudden and unexpected turn.

It was around 8:30 a.m. that autumn day in 1956. I was returning home from my midnight shift at the Secretary of State's office. I had barely passed the civil service exam, so I would have to work my way up the ladder for a better job. The air hung dry and smoky. The tree leaves were brilliant shades of gold and took flight in the sky. The elm tree branches drooped under the enchantment of the leaves. Like the twelve chosen spies sent to search the land of Canaan, the twelve doctors at the University of Michigan Hospital in Ann Arbor, Michigan, were diagnosing my husband Bob's lung condition as terminal.

These are strong words to make peace with. Like sand sifted over and over through a screen, our few alternatives were sifted and weighed carefully. Bob often said that during these hospital stays, his caregivers had control of his body. Filling out forms to be sure insurance would cover the bill; there were endless tests to be evaluated. Seldom was the news good.

Let's turn to the story of Caleb and Joshua to help us.

The spies report to Israel

> And they came and went…unto the wilderness of Paran to Kadesh… and moreover we saw the children of Anak there.
>
> The Amalekites dwell in the land of the south and the Hittes and the Jebusites and the Amorites dwell in the mountains and the Canaanites dwell by the sea.
>
> And there we saw the giants, the son of Anak, which come of the giants. In spite of the giants, Caleb and Joshua gave good reports that the land could be taken.
>
> —Numbers 13:26–33

At this time, it had seemed theoretically possible to start building our three-bedroom country bungalow when Bob suddenly became ill. Now, after picking my two-year-old up from the babysitters', I would head for the University of Michigan Hospital in Ann Arbor to hear the doctor's reports. The two contractors reported they could start building the house as soon as we got the report from the twelve or so specialists regarding how long Bob would be laid up and what effect that would have on our income.

Except for the wind that moved gently through the trees, it was quiet as little Stephen Cooper and I drove along. I found the entrance to the massive hospital with little trouble since I had been there several times to visit Bob. This visit would be different from the others, however, because I would be getting the full report from the diagnostic team.

Bob's bronchial tubes were narrowing and this needed to be treated. It was difficult for air to enter his lungs. His diagnosis was bronchial emphysema. The emphysema would allow his lungs to inflate but not retract. As the result, more and more air was trapped. There was the non-stop rhythm of coughing and wheezing as air tried to force its way through the narrowing air passages to his lungs.

The report certainly was not a good one. The bad report by the Israelite spies said there were too many giants in the Land of Canaan. Bob and I felt like there were many giants in our lives, but we tackled them one at a time. Bob was home on disability for a while, but then returned to his job. The house went up and in the spring of 1957, we moved into the two rooms of the house we had finished and paid for. It took five years to complete the rest of the house but we were debt free, the deed was clear.

Israel refuses to enter Canaan

> And all the congregation lifted up their voices and cried and the people wept that night. All the children of Israel murmured against Moses.
>
> —NUMBERS 14:1–2

I murmured against the doctors from then on.

The bad report of the spies was not as significant as Caleb and Joshua's reaction to it. The Israelites lacked faith in God's promise that He would help them possess the land. Trying to save the day, Caleb and Joshua stepped forward and asked the people to go and possess the land. Bob and my house contractors stepped forward to start our house in hopes of alleviating our sense of despair. Caleb and Joshua were so passionate in their testimony about the taking of the land that they emotionally tore their clothes. The people were not impressed by their emotions. Caleb and Joshua believed the Canaanites' self-absorption and blind wickedness were their weaknesses.

We had a child, and we had to move forward. We praised God when the two carpenters reported that they could finish by winter. This gave us hope.

Now with the passion of the Lord, Caleb and Joshua could have gathered those who would follow them and strike out on their own to take Canaan, but God had a different plan. They would go forth as a congregation. In Numbers 14:24 God did promise Caleb and all his descendants special land in Canaan as a reward for his good report. Caleb believed the promise, so he abided until God again opened the door to possess the land.

Bob and I abided for many years as new medications prolonged his life. The time between the bad report and the end of Bob's life was twelve years. Whereas the time before the Israelites could receive the land was forty years. Bob beat the odds by seven years! I did not divorce Bob as the burdens grew, though it was on my mind from time to time. To me, Bob was justified by faith, was obedient to God, and was a wonderful father. I was his wife and remained faithful and satisfied. Caleb was also satisfied that the alternative course that God set out for all the people would come. Caleb gave up his right to be right so he could stay with the assembly that God wanted brought to the Promised Land.

Now let's look at Elijah. God showed signs of wonder through Elijah, who demonstrated unswerving belief. Then Elijah was attacked by the devil in a weak moment after showing that his God was more powerful then the god Baal (see 1 Kings 19:4). Even though Bob and I saw God was more powerful than Bob's disease, fear gripped us when our little boy became terribly sick with allergies.

Bob also had many bouts with asthma. Ironically, it was our mutual understanding of each other's struggles with asthma that had spurred us to explore other common grounds and led to our marriage in 1950. Our son, Stephen, was born with asthmatic tendencies that caused him much discomfort, especially when we were on the farm where we lived part of the time.

After we were married, Bob farmed large areas of land to insure our dairy farm success. Each morning and evening in the winter he would shovel hay into feeding stalls for the animals, leaving a trail of dust fouled air behind him. Like many farmers, Bob was a hard worker and would care for the animals even though he had a cold, bronchitis or walking pneumonia. Bob gave up farming and went to work at Oldsmobile's Part's Department. After he was hospitalized and given the bad report, he did not want to conceive any more children because he did not want them to develop his condition. Steve had already developed allergies.

Each day that Bob was exposed to more bad air from the factory when he returned to work there, his life expectancy was shortened. Unable to avoid the primary problem of foul factory air, we took control over those areas of our lives affecting the quality of our health that we could control. We examined different food additives and decided to grow our own organic gardens. We froze our harvest and bought our beef directly from farmers who processed non-commercially.

Still, during his bouts of extreme respiratory distress, these processes seemed to bring little relief. It was frightening and frustrating when new tests only confirmed further deterioration. Where could we find relief?

One Sunday, a friend and I visited a Free Methodist church, the denomination of my youth. I reached out to God in my despair and was rewarded with a relationship right with God. Later, in a desperate hour when Bob seemed to no longer be able breath, he asked that I call my pastor. The man of God came right over and Bob gave his life to the Lord. From then on, Bob had his Bible to lean on and I could see signs of hope in his eyes. By giving up his right to be right, to want to live above all else, he found new life in Christ.

I became somewhat dependent on the pastor who counseled me. Dependency is not uncommon where there are caregivers, spiritual or otherwise. This tendency is particularly strong when helping the victims and their families to deal with the trauma. A certain amount of trust or dependency is needed in the therapeutic process. Once the victim learns to trust the therapist, he/she may become somewhat dependent. If one providing the care also has a strong need for someone to depend upon him/her, the environment is ripe for codependency.

For a while, Bob didn't need me quite so often to rub his back and wipe perspiration from his brow after terrible coughing spells. Even the need for emergency medicine lessened in frequency for a time. Bob stopped feeling like he was bashing his heart against the wall, but I began to feel like I was perched on a church steeple again, looking down at the various avenues that all led to one place: Bob's death. Bob, on the other hand, embraced new hope. Over time Bob had learned that, in respect to death, all Christians are promised eternal life in Christ—where there will be no illness, pain, or death.

By 1958, our family needed both our incomes. I had a permanent job at the Secretary of State's Department. I was a case manager for drunk drivers. Providing care for a terminally ill husband, who still had to help with the bread winning, left me with feelings of insecurity. Bob's outlook of the future changed because of the saving power of Jesus Christ. He began setting short-term goals like taking classes in real estate. Bob was a smart man and having the chance to earn good grades and eventually passing the Real Estate Board Exam did great things for his self-esteem.

Many have noted the stages that a person with a terminal illness experiences. I will mention them as they relate to Bob's illness. Denial is common, as is bargaining with God, doctors, spouses, and anyone who could potentially change the final outcome. Both of these are necessary to the coping process. Bob carried inward anger that manifested in explosive outbursts during the most desperate of times. We both fought depression. The fifth stage that terminally ill individuals hopefully attain is resolve. Bob and I found resolve in Jesus Christ. To us, the Christian resolve was the beginning of a new reality in Christ.

The final reaction to pending death is the desire to avoid further pain without the "what ifs." Bob never got to that point. He fought to the very end. He kept limited options open and remained flexible so as not to miss a reasonable strategy that could work to create a new plan of action. He also worked on projects that could be completed in a relatively short amount of time. Bob completed the new house the kitchen cabinets, wearing a dust mask. In his fragile state he put trim around the doors and window in the evening after he finished work. He found working with wood restful. With Bob's real estate license framed on our living room wall, Bob was ready to sell real estate part-time. He was driven, a workaholic. Soon he was making sales but could not always make it to the property closing meetings.

He showed great confidence in me by handing me the book used in his real estate class and telling me to memorize everything in the book so I could pass the real estate exam without having to pay tuition for the class. Remembering my dyslexia, I thought he was nuts, but it worked nevertheless. I sledged through the book and passed the adjusted test. It was hard to give up the job security of my regular job to help Bob, but my involvement in this with him lifted his spirits and gave him hope that there was still a future for him.

We found a house in town on a busy corner where we could eventually include a real estate broker's office. For supplemental income, we also rented out the country home we owned debt-free. With these small steps, using the resources available, I could help meet the needs of our family.

We were aware that our ultimate success depended on God. "The horse is made ready for battle, but victory rests with the Lord" (Prov. 21:31, NIV).

At about this time, I really established myself as a follower of Christ. The warming of the spirit in my soul was indescribable. I knew Jesus was mine and that God had drastically changed the direction of my life. I was called to full-time ministry when I was 28-years-old. I started religious education classes by correspondence, and an opportunity to start a neighborhood *Good News Club* through the *Child Evangelism Fellowship* opened up.

Seemingly all of a sudden, I was carrying the gospel to many churches. Souls were being saved through the weekly outreach program at our church. However, Bob's health was deteriorating. He spent weekends at his mother's house across the road from the farm we owned. Bob was evaluated at the University of Michigan Hospital in Ann Arbor. He learned his life expectancy with emphysema was limited, but steroids were being developed that could lessen his nighttime coughing episodes that were beginning to weaken him greatly. Still, trips to the emergency room for breathing treatments increased. He worried about time slipping away from him. At times he was so ill that I did his brokerage paperwork. He eventually coaxed me into selling homes during the week. In our religious life, I became a guest children's speaker at churches around Michigan on Sunday.

I felt torn, but knew it was right to follow my husband's lead. However, between ministry and real estate, I was putting in about 80 hours a week. Bob still worked full-time (as his health allowed) at General Motors because the health insurance package they offered was essential. Even while juggling work at the factory and in real estate, he still worked toward turning rooms of our townhome into an office.

Prior to my faith renewal and call to Christian service, Bob and I decided to adopt a child. We contacted the probate court and agreed to keep a foster child until a baby became available for adoption. A very ill baby crossed our paths and we cared for him while the doctors restored his health. He became available for adoption and we were elated at the possibility. Stephen, our own son, was five years old at the time; *this precious little infant could complete our family.*

To our devastation; however, something went wrong in the adoption process and the adoption papers were not finalized. The child, now over a year old, would go back to his biological parents who had abused him. The county believed they had been rehabilitated after receiving education and the young parents were thought to be able to take better care of this child.

When that disappointment was behind us, the door opened for me to be active in Christian service that stretched beyond caring for Bob. Once we begin thinking of needs of the flesh over spiritual needs, our judgment falters. I did not think a premonition I had about Bob's death was a warning to cut back on some responsibilities so I could deal with the loss I would feel after Bob's death.

Then, a temptation was placed before me. A five-year-old girl named Sue was available for adoption. We consulted Bob's doctors. They would place no guarantee, but ten more years of life was possible with careful planning. Our life was already complicated enough, but the desire to escape the boring routine of Bob's hospital stays and household responsibilities prevailed. We did not realize that when daily life already has too many duties, bringing a child of any age into our world only complicates matters. We believed our desires were from the Holy Spirit.

We found out that we could have this little girl by Christmas Day of 1962. A fresh and positive outlook toward the future was opened to us; *this would take our minds off Bob's health.* We did not allow ourselves to think of how demanding small children could be, and the caseworker had not disclosed to us that Sue would need extra adjustment time.

I assumed this child's giggles would fill my need for a quick fix to brighten my day–*I could just give her a hug, and she would give me one in return.*

Rather than being healthy enough myself to raise a child with challenges, I was looking to her to fulfill my emotional need—distract me from the trying issues in my life.

Despite bouts in the hospital and working full-time, Bob studied and passed the State of Michigan Brokers examination. We felt like we were on top of everything.

With another child now in our home, the responsibility of walking out my God-given anointing for church ministry was faltering. The time I had to prepare for teaching Christian education slipped; I could not keep up the pace. God gave me my little girl, but allowed the anointing of ministering to people beyond my family, friends, and business associates slip away. He loved me and knew my limits even if I didn't.

The beautiful, blue-eyed, five-year-old had been my Christmas gift of 1963. Her new father, brother, and I loved her right away. Professionals told us that her hyperactive behavior and school adjustment problems could be explained by the fact that she had been moved from the last of many foster homes in the middle of the school year and was adjusting to having a new name and family.

Her social worker told us that she was from an abusive home. Nothing was explained to us; we did not know what this really meant. When our caseworker told us "our love would heal all," we believed it. So, a year and a half later she became our little girl by adoption.

To our dismay, her problems persisted and on the advice of our physician we arranged for some medical tests, including a brain test. Our medical doctor's suspicions were confirmed—she had a brain injury either by birth or accident. The school staff advised us that a program for the emotionally disturbed was the answer. But lost in a sea of what seemed to us to be appropriate school-advised therapy, our frustrations and fears for her future kept us emotionally drained as years filled with worsening learning and behavioral problems passed.

When she was thirteen years old, there was no junior high school program geared for her in our city. Therefore, the school professionals advised us to take her out of our nurturing arms and place her in a structured home for girls. We trusted them, so with tears in our eyes and a feeling of failure, we took her to the appointed city where the girl's home and school program were located. This program for the emotionally disturbed seemed even more difficult for her adjustment problems. Although physically exhausted, we made the trip to the neighboring city to visit her as much as possible even though Bob's health was failing in an extreme way now and we were also dealing with demands of full-time jobs (Stephen worked part-time while in high school).

Five months passed, then in January of 1971, just when it seemed Sue was responding a little to her new surroundings, her father and my first husband died. She screamed, "My Daddy's dead," as she fled from the room when she was told. Dark days followed. At her resident girl's home, there was so much structure, I believe she needed Stephen's and my daily support. We three needed to work through her grief together but it was not possible.

Our little girl had as much instability as her young life could stand. She began to run away. Though vulnerable to every kind of street predator, she tried to make her own way.

Difficult decisions had to be made. State-funded mental health services would be available to save her under the state's care.

The plan didn't work.

Years later, still lost to me, my son, and society, we have no idea of her whereabouts.

Now that I can recognize and better understand the behavior patterns that are characteristic of many brain-injured individuals, it is not uncommon for me to see the face of my little girl in theirs. When I see other brain-injured individuals improving as the result of well targeted and fully understood programs for the brain-injured, it is like a little part of her has been salvaged. Only then does she no longer seem lost to me. I cannot help but search the crowds looking for her sky blue eyes and flying hair.

God does not waste any ability we have. All gifts can be useful to Him, even if we learned them by default. Sue showed key ADHD characteristics that were similar to my yet undiagnosed ADHD. Years later in my second marriage when my adopted son David developed ADHD from his injury, I finally understood that his and Sue's behaviors were similar and that David was not just being uncooperative as others' had thought. Learning this was a start, a beginning point, for me in my discovery of how to help other caregivers gain the coping skill of not that will dwelling on the fact that our lives do not always turn out the way we would have chosen. This was a lesson that I had gleaned early from my father, my caregiver who had taught me that there are times when life take difficult turns and families just have to let go of "what could have been" and abide as happily and peacefully in "what now is." However, burying what we cannot deal with is not the answer. It will only resurface with another face.

I was not emotionally prepared for Bob's death. I fell into what some call a "spiritual black hole." This happens when our inner life in Christ is neglected. In my life, I thought less and less about making full-time Christian service my vocation. I wanted a replacement husband to share my life. How could I go it alone? I thought my dreams could be seen as godly purposes, and that included my new fantasies to marry. My children needed a father.

I was thirty-nine years old and needed a husband. I was not entirely leaving that which God had called me to, but I rationalized that I would do it part-time. It would not be the complete will of God, but I sensed that it would be the will of God for me to marry again.

Many Christians do serve for Christ without the anointing (God's calling on ones on whom is His power to act.) In the Bible, Paul said that if a widow could not control her passion, she should marry again. I would marry a Christian, and the idea surfaced that that would please God; but we cannot tell God what will please Him. Things are more complicated than that and the Lord would have a lot to show me, both from failures and from triumphs during the course of my second marriage.

I was like Caleb when he trotted along with those who had listened to the false reports about insurmountable obstacles to taking Canaan. I had followed my first husband Bob and God blessed our limitations to the point where we were making a good living. But when he died, I was like Elijah was after he had experienced the high of proving to Queen Jezebel and King Ahab that his God was the one and only true God. What faith it took! For Elijah to call fire down from heaven to consume the water-drenched altar of Baal, and thereby win many believers, was amazing! On that high, Satan tempted Elijah at his weakest point, fear. When the wicked Queen Jezebel ordered him killed, Elijah ran and hid in a cave. God fed Elijah and returned him to health. Although he did not trust God and therefore ran from Queen Jezebel, God did not take away his anointing but called him to anoint Elisha as his successor. I believe that when I remarried, God passed my anointing to another for a time.

Was Bob's death a waste? Of course not! When I took him to the hospital in early January of 1971, he was ready to meet his wonderful Maker. This time the emergency breathing treatments did not work. His worn-out heart quit beating.

The loss to my son was enormous. Throughout Stephen Cooper's childhood Bob had made the effort to spend time with his son. Many hours each year were spent hunting and fishing. The two-hour drive they took to Bob's old farm on many weekends had given them much time to talk. Bob was able to pass onto Stephen Cooper his conservative politics, a love for his country, and his strong work ethic. Although my second husband and I played a significant role in helping Stephen Cooper attain goals, Bob had taught him to believe in himself and never give up. There was something else that Bob passed on to Stephen Cooper: an enduring faith in Jesus Christ.

Although Bob passed when our son was only sixteen, Stephen can still call to mind the image of his father quietly reading from his Bible in the evening. In the months just prior to his death, Bob made an extra effort to spend time with him. His lungs were too weak from emphysema to go into the field with him that last year when Bob took Stephen for their fall hunt, but he went as far as he could. In fact, he went as far as he could in all things with Stephen; and in so doing he was quietly preparing him for a future without his father. Stephen Cooper will always cherish the memories of their time together, hunting, fishing, color tours and together enjoying the beauty and majesty of nature. He also remembers his father's values and faith. Bob's act of spending time instructing our son in Bible truths reminds me of the promise Caleb had that his descendents would inherit the Promised Land. We now have great-grandchildren who God is guiding through Christian parenting.

As for me, my journey of restoration would ultimately lead me to the place where I am no longer confused by being afraid of authority figures. Sorting through my past was critical to my roots growing deep in a soil that was not littered by wounds that lingered for too long. This important cleaning of the soil of my heart would bring to the place where I can now move in the discernment of spirits, like Elijah. This discernment now helps me to override some of the symptoms of my thorn in my side—my lifelong personal struggle with ADHD.

I believe the anointing can leave us if we do not, for the sake of God's kingdom, give up the right to be right—much like Caleb and Joshua did. It was not wrong for me to want children and remarry, but the anointing for Christian service left when I threw caution to the wind and chased the Promised Land in my own timing and on my own terms. When I did that God stopped speaking to my soul about Christian service and I believe He began to speak to someone else about what He had had in store for me. Much of what had been planned for me was now dead—to me anyway. I became dead in Christ like Elijah when taken to Heaven. Many years would pass before I heard the gentle words of Jesus say to me, "You are my little Elijah girl again. You have my anointing."

So as to more illustrate my point that God can and will take away the anointing from someone who chooses to trade it for something else, I will take us forward to one day in 1998. I was twenty-six years into my second marriage to Bill when I was invited to a convention center to hear a well-known TV evangelist/teacher. I had listened to several of her book-tapes.

In pretty short order after I found my seat, I was taken back something the evangelist prophesized. "There are older ones here tonight whom God anointed when they were still young that are still under the same anointing and do not know it."

She described how one would know what a true anointing was. As my mind searched the past, I felt like a priceless black diamond that had just begun to sparkle. A camp meeting I had gone to when I was fifteen came to mind. An evangelist, triumphant over Russian persecution that caused him to have only partial use of his legs, picked me out of a crowd of nearly 500 believers and anointed me. He believed God had spoken to him regarding me. He refused assistance and struggled off the platform without struggling, making his way toward me. According to the evangelist, a recipient's knowledge of their anointing is constant and timeless. The one to be anointed would somehow know ahead of time that they were to be anointed.

All those years earlier, that Russian had adamantly refused the use of his wheelchair and inched his way toward me as he pulled himself from one pew to anther. I wanted to run and help him, but I also wanted to slip out through the side curtain. I knew he was coming to me and I could not stop my tears. "Please let him hurry," I prayed. Even though he was clearly in great pain, he was completely obedient to God. When he finally got to me, he placed his hands on my head and prophesized over me. I ran to the altar. There, the Spirit touched me and I began to spin in a circle while on my knees. This behavior was not uncommon at that time in that denomination. Even so, it was the outward expression of the witness of the Spirit.

As I contemplated what the Tele-evangelist had said, I saw a match between her prophecy and what had happened to me that year when I was a teen who was honored by the camp saints during their two-week long gathering. By the time I had gone home from camp, however, my shallow faith had waned and had come away with the belief that it had just been a camp experience.

Hearing that Tele-evangelist's word's caused me take a second look at the anointing from which I had departed when I thought I was too burnt out from care-giving to carry the burdens of daily life on my own while I waited on the Lord for additional direction. In some ways, my marriage to Bill was a refuge for me, a place of refuge where my new husband became my new caregiver. The gifts of God are without repentance and the time would come again when God would ignite my gifts with the fire of the anointing of His Spirit.

Eventually the Lord would begin directing me to public ministry again, but the turn I took in my life would bring new responsibilities and new distractions from my relationship with the Lord.

Even if we have made wrong turns or turned too quickly, God will bring us around the backside of the desert again and give us another

Bill, Jan and David Warrington

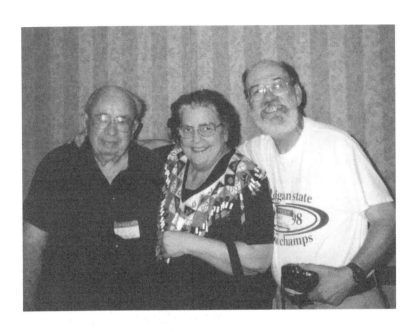

chance to abide in patience and obedience like that of Caleb's. Many times bringing us around again will begin with Him unraveling the tangles of our lives and helping us to build a little altar in our minds to worship Him. I take courage in this when I think of my dear, sweet mother who was the victim of circumstances when she was brain-injured while being treated for simple depression. Even in the bleakest of places and seemingly hopeless of circumstances, she built a little altar of worship for her family right there in the middle of a dingy and decrepit mental institution that afternoon in 1941.

With that in mind, surely we can circle back around to the feet of Jesus. We cannot always be right, but that's okay. God can turn a wrong into a right and give us grace to endure. Simple daily prayer and Bible reading can center our focus on our Maker. Worshiping in our mind allows for commitments to be established and reinforced between God and us.

As I circled around to the feet of Jesus, where I would find the grace to be a mature and whole Christian who walked in the anointing of the Holy Spirit, I also took comfort in knowing that I will see Bob again in Heaven and Bill will see his departed first wife Irene as well.

My Savior was being patient with me and my headaches were staying at bay more and more as the irresistible power of the hand of God within me was gentle, like a surgeon's hand taking out slivers that had festered for a long time without care. It hurt! Oh, how it hurt to let go of bitterness and truly forgive those people and events that had caused (and were still causing) me so much emotional pain.

Bill and Jan, 1972

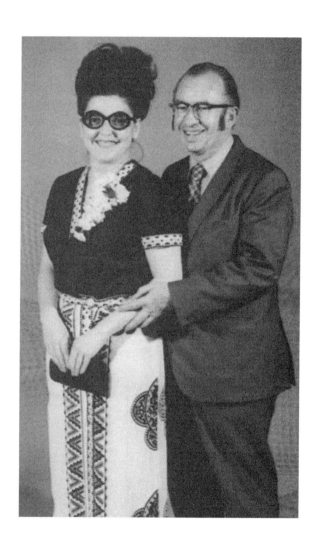

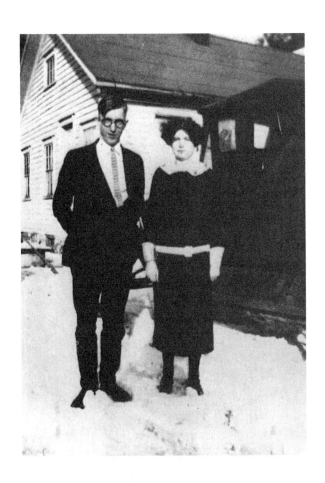

My father and mother

Grandma and Grandpa

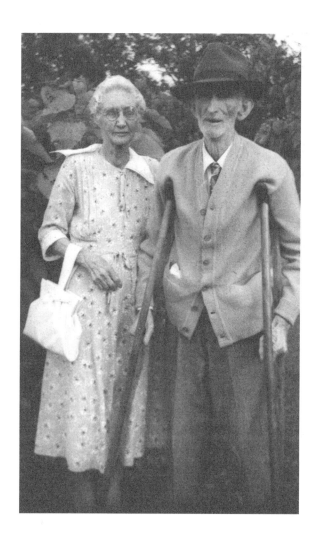

My maternal grandmother

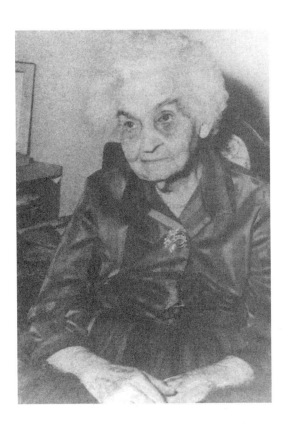

Aunt and uncle I lived with as a child

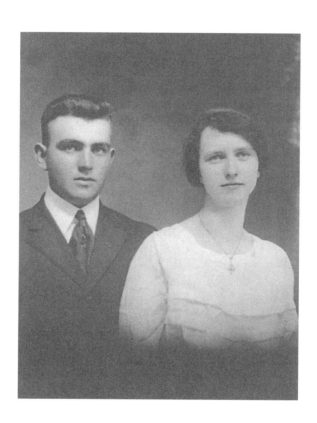

☛ My father and his brother, sister and mother (extended family caregivers; child unknown). Left to right: Doris, John, Rosella, my father, Veda, Harvey, and Marjorie. Grandma is seated. ☚

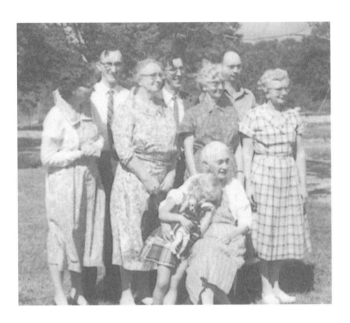

Dr. Willard (Bill) Warrington at his office, 1976.

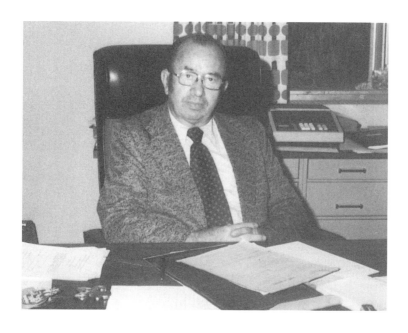

Aunt Marjorie Edwards, my Dad's sister. Extended caregiver, 1960.

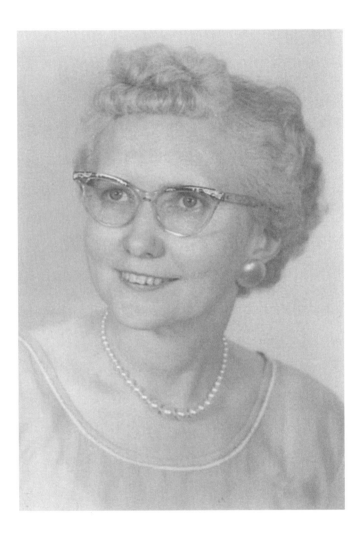

Victory over the mystery house of my childhood.

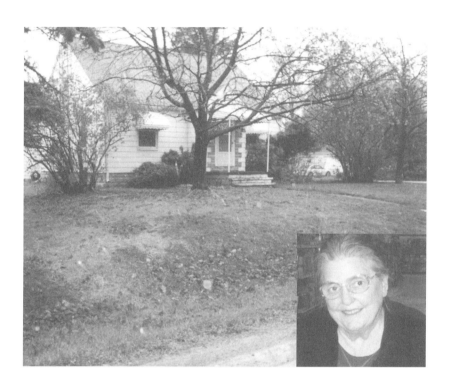

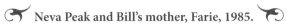 Neva Peak and Bill's mother, Farie, 1985.

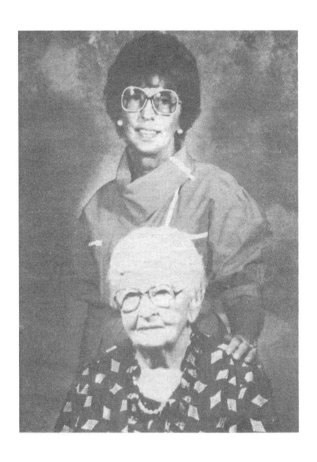

Grandnieces Rebecca and Sara Wyczalek (L-R).

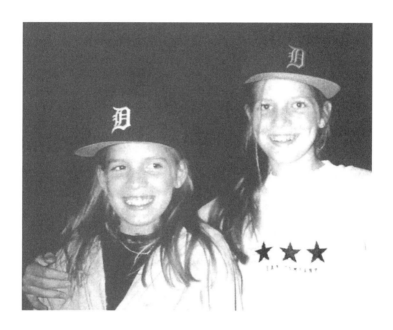

Jan and Bob Cooper, 1950.

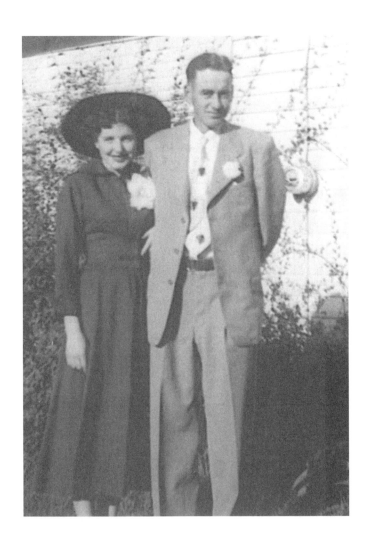

Bonnie and Steve Cooper, 1974.

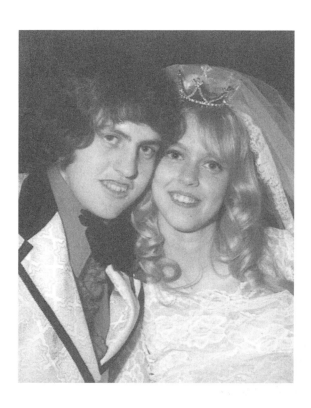

David riding a bike, 1979.

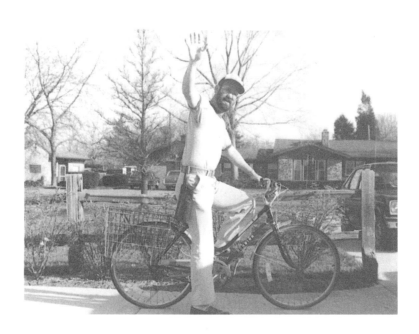

Steven, Katie, and Robert Cooper (top to bottom).

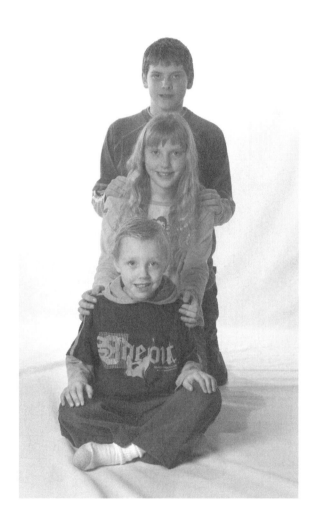

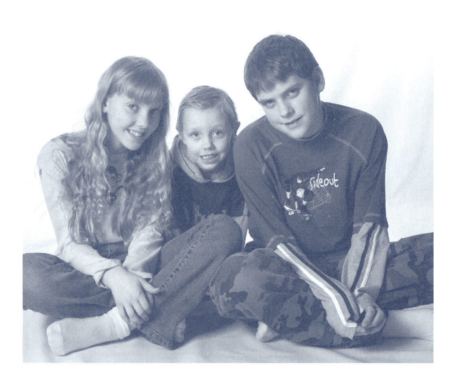

Katie, Robert, and Steven Cooper (L-R).

Robert, Katie, and Steven Cooper, and Jan

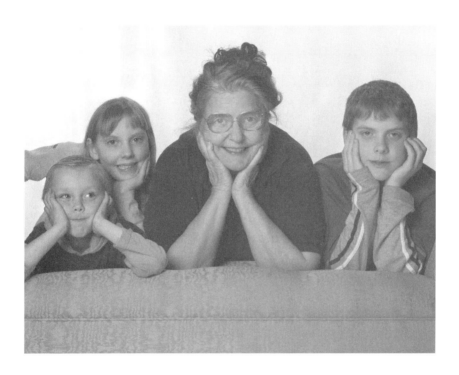

Great-grandchild Evelyn Firman

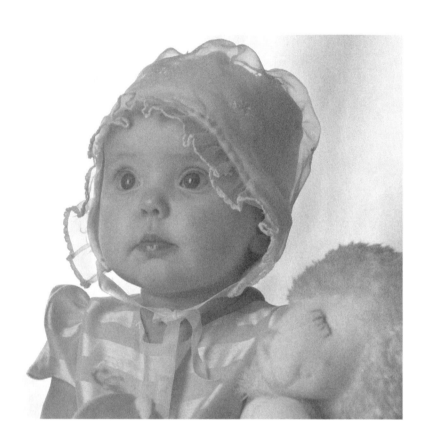

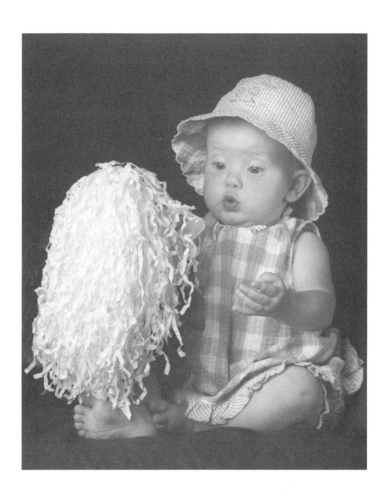

❦ 9 ❧

Grieving Great Losses

I HAD ALREADY LOST my husband Bob that year and Sue was lost to me as well. Now, out of the blue I received a telephone call telling me that my mother was dying from cancer. Would I go see her? Of course I would go. I had not seen my mother since I visited her at the sanitarium in 1950; the year I married Bob. I had no idea what to expect. I told Stephen, then just sixteen, that I was taking him to visit his grandmother. I had never talked to him about my mother. I had only told him that during my formative years I had lived with my parents and brothers and sisters.

I tried to prepare Stephen for the visit. Again, I didn't know what to tell him. Perhaps an emotional rush of ADHD or unanswered grief caused my mind to wander back to my first few visits to see her in the mental hospital. My mind replayed the worst scenarios. I remembered the bleak halls lined with shock treatment patients. I did not see any private rooms, only wards for mental patients. *Perhaps there are private rooms now, with pretty papered walls. What could I say to him?* I finally gave up and told my son to pray to God for understanding.

After explaining to him what had happened, I told him that his grandfather, whom he loved so much, felt it was important to keep a mother figure in the home and told him of the sacrifices we all made to keep Mom there as long as possible, especially when we children were small.

I took my son to see my mother. It must have been on a Sunday, nearly six months after my first husband's death. It was a relief when the nurses told me they were keeping my mother out of pain. Bob had suffered in pain for so long. This unhappy crisis prompted me to tell Stephen what I remembered that was wonderful about my mother. Then I remembered how I went to the neighbors' a lot when I was a child. Dare I now think about what I dared not to think about as a child? We children seemingly could not comprehend Mom's depression as it lay before us on those grim days. My mother's efforts to go through her usual duties, only to stop and cry over past sorrows of a little girl lost to her forever—herself.

We parked the car close by on the day Stephen and I visited Mom. I pulled Stephen to me and kissed him as we walked to the hospital. We found the registration desk and someone took us to her wing. As we slowly walked down the hall, I noticed pretty curtains in the windows and sure enough the walls were papered. Remembering past efforts, I was glad I hadn't done the papering. Still, the hollow clunking of shoes echoed off the same granite floors as my childhood visits. A nurse walked down the hall with us. This place was not my home, yet it was my mother's home for far too many years. Although I was uneasy while waiting to see her, I would respect this place, I would respect my mother's home.

There were only a few patients in the hospital rooms. We were past the 1960's era of mental hospital reform, and many medicated patients were in foster homes or back home with their families. One nurse was worried over the plight of those released who did not have strong enough connections back in their communities to help them. It wasn't pleasing that some of the unwanted or unacceptable were now living on the streets.

(As the image of my mother lying on that bed came to my mind as I was reviewing that heart-wrenching event with the Lord, I realized that her hair was as white as pure spilled sugar. It reminded me of the mountains I saw on the way to Huntersville, Georgia, that wintry holiday season in 1985. I thought of the deer hunt that could have been fun with a spirited partner. My mother had not been my father's partner all these years but on that day in the hospital I had seen her as being both my mother and my partner in Christian faith. The Psalmist tells us of the deer panting for a brook. "As the deer pants for the water brooks, so my soul pants for You, O God" (Psalm 42:1, NAS). Often a predator would chase the deer, panting to reach the brook. The deer could float downstream and the water would wash away its scent so the predator could not follow. Depression had been my mother's predator but now her body and soul seemed to be panting for her home in heaven. Thinking of the spotting of green not hidden by the snow in the Kentucky Mountains reminded me of us children she bore in her young adult years.)

As Stephen and I took turns explaining our positive successes in life, we could not tell if she sensed how we were an extension of her that can live on. We five living children were like the strength of the mountain that stood so high against the winds of life. Softly and quietly she breathed, her chest moving up and down. She looked squarely at me. In response to her look, I said, "This is your grandson, Stephen."

Maybe, maybe, maybe, echoed in my mind and I repeated it under my breath. "Why am I doing this?" I thought. In that moment it seemed nothing had changed since I was a child when she would only answer "Maybe" when I so desperately needed her.

The insecurities of "maybe" were far too often in my lifetime. *God, help me and mine.* I forced myself to control my emotions. My mother had been sick for years and I had not been at her side. I only knew I loved her and wanted to be near her that day and many, many days before. Oh, so many before.

> Behold, she is like my mountain. Her feet brought good tidings and she proclaimed peace! God, in waiting, has her feast. She performed her vows young; for the pain shall no more pass.

I kissed my mother. Her room was warm and inviting with comfortable chairs. She looked me over head-to-toe, with the strangest look on her face, as if she was looking over a newborn baby. I had told her who I was, but whether she knew, I'll never know. What could she have been thinking?

As I reviewed this in my mind before the Lord, I suddenly I realized what has been at the heart of much of my anger and fear: I had been suffering from feelings of abandonment. First, by my mother and then by my first husband, Bob, and finally by a child I believed I had failed.

I also realized that I had remorse over having not been by my mother's side and not having tried to get her out of the hospital. And could it be that I was angry at my father for discouraging me from going to see her? I didn't want to think about these things, but I had to face emotional and spiritual pain so I could be free of the physical pain of the headaches. As I relayed this in my mind, I prayed that God would help me with each emotion that surfaced as I walked through each corner of my memory, took the contents off of the shelf, examined it before the Lord, and put it back on the shelf that God and I shared—the shelf of peace in Jesus Christ.

A nurse came in and tried to bridge the gap. "She can talk," the nurse explained to me, "but she had a stroke that caused her to slur her words."

The nurse reaffirmed to my mother who I was. Tears filled my eyes when I couldn't understand a question my mother asked. Since I was a very small child, I had yearned for her voice to instruct me, to answer my questions, to show me the way through the valleys of life; now she was responding and I could not understand her. Please, God, help me to understand what she is saying. I turned my head so she could not see my anguish. Esther, a friend of ours, had been a nurse at the hospital. She knew my mother while working there. She said my mother had asked about her children, but my father never encouraged us to visit. Had he given up? Why?

My mother passed away quietly soon after.

My family gathered for my mother's funeral at a sibling's house; some flying in from different parts of the country. There were so many unanswered questions and memories to share. At the graveside, a sibling took her husband's arm and my dad took mine. He cried, "I want my girl." He showed so much love for my mother after all these years; it was amazing.

My father never remarried. (As I thought about my parents' love for one another while I brought this painful experience before the Lord, I thought of how my parents believed that Grace and Sovereignty cannot be questioned, and we all may understand the magnitude of God's caregiving power by the sheer fact that my father was still alive after his encounter with the man with the axe. I believe God intervened. I also believe God used both my mother and my father's faith in those moments that could have snuffed out his life.)

Hot tears flowed down my face as we sat next to her casket at the cemetery that warm day of remembrance and closure of a life. I emerged from the funeral cherishing the better memories exchanged between my family members. We were still a family, and our children all romped with one another and greeted each other warmly at family reunions. I love my family and all they have accomplished. Yes, the hunt was really for my mother. I saw her in my child and nieces and nephews. Their hair and eyes are like hers and they have warm personalities and a sense of humor like hers. My sisters look like her, also. I look like my dad, but I have her coloring. My brothers have her humor.

Looking back as I write this account, I can now associate my mother's death and her characteristics seen in her offspring when I think of Christ's death and resurrection making it possible, through the Holy Spirit, for others to see Christ-like characteristics in us. I am also comforted in the fact that she can be seen in me and in others who make up her legacy.

Mother's death that summer made us all have sorrowful hearts. Yet I could not share my grief while I was trying to adjust to losses. We gathered at one of my family member's homes after my mother's funeral. People we had known all our life saw the obituary and came to the funeral home.

On the way, my mind had raced again over my earlier life, trying to get rid of my pain. When, as a child, I started making the rounds of the neighborhood was I trying to escape what I dare not feel, sense what I dare not sense? Yes, my life, as I knew it then, was crumbling before me. I must get away! I was reliving it. My mother again crumbled before me, with barely a word spoken between us. She had to have known I was her daughter, or I cannot bare it. But I will see her in heaven.

As I took this painful experience to the Lord much in the way that you would stop and start a movie that was playing in my mind, I grieved deeply before the Lord. I would later learn that my running was probably a combination of escaping the pain at home and also a symptom of ADHD with a bout of Obsessive Compulsive Disorder that was manifesting under great stress.

🔸 10 🔸

Picking Up the Pieces

A s I CONTINUED to leave behind and learn from the wounds of the past and to re-glean what God had given me in those past events, I knew my journey toward being more whole and more like Christ was edging me closer and closer to the fresh wounds of not so long ago.

At the grief class I attended after my first husband Bob had passed, it was suggested that I try their singles' social group. It was there that I met, fell in love and married my wonderful Bill. On that day, April 26, 1972, I started a brighter path. My caring husband, Bill, continues to look after our whole family, as his age and strength and our children and their families permit.

You may want to know a little about what my husband is like. A poem read in worship can give truth that may be hard to express otherwise. Generally known historical poets were some of the first to be killed in revolutions because of truths expressed within their thoughts on paper. Carl Moll, who resides in a retirement park we lived in, wrote the following portion of a poem about Bill.

JUST PLAIN BILL

Every once in a while a man comes along
That stands out in his willingness to show
Though not necessarily physically strong
He's intellectually firm in the know
A man who always stands ready to give
But who offers only when asked

A sturdy citizen of character willing to live
Quietly ready whatever the task
Only on rare occasions when a snag or stall
Threatens to cause an unnecessary bicker
This man will stand up, this man will stand tall
And in a few words unravel the kicker

We are much richer for having her here
His counsel an ever steadying force
I know he's not looking for praise or a cheer
He'd say he doesn't deserve it of course

No one asked me to do this but I must
I hereby without hesitation
Before I end up where dust turns to dust
Let's put an end to procrastination
Mr. Warrington who prefers just Bill
It with great pride I call you my friend.

—Carl Moll

Life was so full of ugliness at the time I married Bill. I yearned to connect with someone when I found Bill. As we each showed our pain to each other, we found love and married in April of 1972. We embraced each other rather than making judgments. Our marriage has lasted thirty-two years. We love each other deeply.

Noted psychologist Carl Rogers suggests there is no atonement needed when two people can connect. Bill and I connected, but our Christian beliefs were different, so we gave and took with each other and concentrated on our worship commonalties. At times it was hard not to become complacent and turn our attention to other solutions such as David's long road to find more meaningful living.

Growing With David

Our son, David, was given back the gift of life. A week after David began coming out of his coma from his brain injury, Bill and I said a prayer with our pastor. This included taking part in a private communion of bread and wine. The pastor, Bill, and I placed David in God's healing hands, to make him whole as He saw fit.

We learned later that the day after our private prayer and healing session our son Douglas, now deceased, had visited David. Something unexpected happened. Douglas called me from David's room very excited. "Jan," he said, "David is talking."

"He's talking! I can't believe it!" I said.

"Yes, he's making sense. It's not just random numbers and phrases. He's responding to me," Douglas replied.

"How did it happen, Douglas?" I asked.

"Well I simply asked him if he could talk, and he said yes. So I suggested we discard the finger method we were using to communicate— one finger up for "yes"; two fingers up "no"—and start talking, and David said 'Okay.'"

I quickly called Bill who was so relieved by the good news. We do not have to discard finger methods or any other ways of communicating to get a hold of God. We cry out and He hears.

> I can do all things through Christ who strengthens.
> —PHILIPPIANS 4:13, RSV

Nothing goes to Heaven surer than Charity, and nothing is so fit to sit in Heaven. Paul had many things to be proud of and to praise in himself-things that the world is more apt to admire than Christian charity, the sweetest, but humblest of all the Christian graces. Paul, I say, was a bulwark of learning, an anchor of faith, a rock of constancy, a thunderbolt of zeal; yet see how he bestows the palm. Could Bill and I show this kind of charity when we tried to help David along with all of our family?

> If I could speak in any language in Heaven and or on earth, but did not love others, I would only be making meaningless noise like a loud gong or a clanging cymbal. If I had the gift of prophecy, and if I knew all the mysteries of the future and knew everything about everything, but didn't love others, what good would I be? And if I had the gift of faith so that I could speak to a mountains and make it move, without love I would be no good to anybody. If I gave everything I have to feed the poor and even sacrificed my

body, I could boast about it; but if I didn't love others, I would be of no value whatsoever.

Love is patient and kind. Love is not jealous or boastful or proud or rude. Love does not demand its own way. Love is not irritable, and it keeps no record of when it has been wronged. It is never glad about injustice but rejoices whenever the truth wins out. Love never gives up, never loses faith, is always hopeful, and endures through every circumstance/

Love will last forever, but prophecy and speaking in unknown languages and special knowledge will all disappear. Now we know only a little, and even the gift of prophecy reveals little! But when the end comes, these special gifts will all disappear.

It is like this: When I was a child, I spoke and thought and reasoned like a child. But when I grew up, I put away childish things. Now we see things imperfectly as in a poor mirror, but then we will see everything with perfect clarity. All that I know now is partial and incomplete, but then I will know everything completely, just as God knows me now.

There are three things that will endure–faith, hope, and love–and the greatest of these is love.

—1 Corinthians 13:1–13, RSV

After David's accident, Bill and I threw ourselves into the fray of caring for him. Where our adrenaline came from, I'm not sure. It surely was from God, likened unto my dad when he was trying to hold our family together during the 1930's depression. No one could do what we were doing for David with love as the pusher for any length of time.

A brain-injured patient may not show behavioral changes in the structured environment of the hospital or rehabilitation facility, but we saw changes in David as soon as he was out of his coma. At home our family saw more changes as soon as David returned to our family environment.

We as a family experienced bewilderment, self-doubt, denial, anger and concern. I believe we needed to have someone who could assist us in working through our feelings. Someone more qualified than those whom we had available to us as at the time.

Earlier, David started seeing a local, highly recommended clinical psychologist who worked with brain-injured people. We had no idea how much the psychologist would be able to help David because we were never able to discuss or learn from him what David talked to him about. Sometimes when we asked David, he would say, "Most of the time we just talked sports—the latest football or basketball scores." Of course, during this period when he had so few friends, we felt that if the psychologist did nothing else, he could at least be a friend to David.

Starting in October 1975, David and I went to a ceramics class weekly. Because it was so far from our home, it was easier for me to attend the class with him than to make two round trips. I decided to do a ceramics project myself; and for David's sake, I became a participant in the group rather than waiting and making him feel it was only appropriate for "crazy club people," as he described it. There were many in the class just because they enjoyed ceramics. I was able to point this out to him.

In 1975, when dealing with David, he vocalized he was in agony with an itch he felt but we could not see, along with his claim that one beer made him drunk. Hospital staff confirmed that this can happen with the brain injured, so in David's case it was true. We learned not to ignore information he gave, no matter how incorrect it seemed, for it often helped us define the problem. The itch was treated and he now stays away from beer and other forms of alcohol. The search for the solutions to the wave-like problems of David's recovery continued.

Once after Bill observed David at a ceramics project, Bill abruptly said he wanted us to leave quietly and return when class was over. When we got in the car, he put his head down on the steering wheel and sobbed. I told Bill we did not have to leave David in the ceramics class if he didn't think it was right for him. "That's not the problem," he said. "To have an outlet for some of his loud behaviors without undue correcting, this is exactly where he should be."

Following a rehabilitation counselor's advice, David became involved daily in a variety of activities like the successful ceramics class, and other educational, social, and recreational challenges. Later, a neurophysiologist agreed. Specific recommendations were also made, such as a remedial reading class, comparable with that which David was taking at Michigan State University and the regular counseling from a private psychologist.

Because of David's educational background, he was permitted to read doctors' reports to help him become more aware of his predicament at this point in his rehabilitation. His reaction was, "When will I be able to return to teaching?" Testing could not provide this information. We heard various opinions from experts, including no recovery after a year or even two years, and more commonly, a prediction of three years. It was no wonder David wanted some hard facts about the likely results of the extensive therapy recommended.

In the book *Feeling and Healing Your Emotions* by Conrad W. Baars, MD, the author asks the rhetorical question, "What are the more specific symptoms of the obsessive compulsive behavior?"[1] It could have appeared we showed temporary bouts of compulsive behavior. In the early days of David's 1975 brain-injury accident, Bill and I would hold it together at work; but when he came home, we both showed temporary bouts of compulsive, ritualistic behavior. For example, in the middle of getting ready for important appointments, discussions, or functions, we would have the household go on hunting sprees to find some simple item like the blue handled tack hammer instead of the handy black one. I use the telephone compulsively to straighten out matters when letter and appointment making could be more appropriate. I still have to work at it for change.

We had so little control over David's problems. At times, without realizing it, we searched for something that could stay stable in one place, like insisting a tack hammer sit on the fireplace mantel. This behavior had to change before all our support systems abandoned us. Every moment was so crammed with thoughts of David, we could not sort out how to even begin to settle down and do anything else. At times we seemed to run from crisis to crisis out of control.

David was tested for cognitive abilities along with attention span deficit and hyperactive behaviors. The test reports provided us with some direction and support for the plan of action we had developed for David's rehabilitation.

David used humor in difficult situations before the accident. Now when his father asked David about his behavior, he would answer, "I was negligent," even when he was not.

David's final words in the matter were, "Jan, it would make me feel better if you would just wear your watch." A ritualistic answer David used a lot. We laughed, hoping the hard crust David had built between himself and me had been broken down.

Before his brain injury, our David was always in the middle of struggles and activities that affected him, his friends, and colleagues. He was very liberal in his political views, participating in peace marches and protests.

He was sometimes very sarcastic and cynical, striking out a conversation in almost any form. Sometimes, if he had to work with conservative people—"straights" as he called them—he would ignore them. He did not say rude things to them; they just were not there. Although he often bought and wore second-hand clothes by preference, he was not gaudy but neat and tidy in appearance.

God reminded me that other brain injured family members were worse off. Some of their children had brain injuries as well as spinal cord severing. Pity parties were not the answer. Prayer was.

A consumer's viewpoint

Where doors are shut, continuing to dialog may help. My grandson attends a Christian school but takes speech improvement classes at a public school. Many Christian colleges and universities provide assistance to all kinds of ably challenged individuals. Paraplegics may differ according to their challenges. Less obvious, but similar, some individuals with learning disorders such as dyslexia may do fine in a classroom without special consideration where others at lower levels may not. Hence the Bible says to do all things without argument or dispute. This can be difficult for caregivers who provide help for the ably challenged in spite of hardship.

One hot day David used poor judgment when he bought the two of us a double-dip ice cream cone without first being sure that he knew where we had parked. It took too much time for him to find the car. By the time he reached it, the ice cream cones were a melted disaster—all down his legs and even into his shoes. I prayed to God for patience.

With this renewed faith, I said quietly to David, "I'm so glad you found the car. It must have been so very hard for you on such a hot day and with two ice cream cones, too!" David agreed and I asked if he saw anyone else having this problem. He thought a moment, then, somewhat bewildered, answered, "No, I didn't. I wonder how other people manage ice cream on such a hot day." "Do you suppose they might just buy one scoop of ice cream?" I hinted. David responded, "Could be." I then suggested that maybe they ate their ice cream in the air-conditioned store; or if they wanted more than one dip, perhaps they ate one dip inside the store and one outside.

As David continued to tell me about the wonderful selections the store had, I gathered up tissues to clean him off. I wrapped the tissues around the cones and somehow started for home, thanking him for the ice cream. I wanted to scream, yell, and bang my head through the solid wall he projected. If only I could escape from the car and run until exhausted, I thought. But that didn't make sense. If only I could shock him into changing by saying, "David, you are a teacher. How do you ever hope to teach again?" Yet all David could understand was that he had found the car successfully. He would be hurt if I didn't like his refreshing gift.

A prayer began to form in my mind. It was to be my guide from then on through all my ordeals with David: Dear God, it takes courage to live one's life and to help others find the courage to live theirs. So many protests! Why should I have the courage when no one understands the sense of outrage life has beset upon me?

One day David and I went to a mall missionary station for directions on how to get to a hotel we were looking for. The missionary singer wanted to tell us about his faith along with directions. I explained that David might not remember any commitment that he might make to the cause.

David felt I was insulting his intelligence. Infuriated, he was determined to listen to the missionary. Because of David's verbal ability and his appearance of well being, the young missionary had no reason to believe he did not have a potential convert.

I knew that I could not talk David out of this conversation. I sat on the couch nearby cooling my heels. David agreed with everything he heard. As a Christian, I was not against what they were doing, but I was doubtful that David, at this stage in his recovery, could be a valid convert. I had not been able to convey this to the young man. David signed a commitment card of some kind. I thought we would be on our way. Instead, a young man with a guitar asked David if he would like to sing a song of religious praise.

I found a magazine and buried my head in it, not wanting to become involved. I knew what would follow. The young guitarist asked David if he knew any religious songs. David said he did not. Then his eyes lit up. "I know 'Bringing in the Cheese!'" he exclaimed. David could not master the true title, "Bringing in the Sheaves."

"'Bringing in the Cheese' I'm not sure I know that one."

"It's a religious song," David said.

The guitarist paused. "Why don't you start the song and maybe we can join in," he said.

David started in a fine singing voice, "Bringing in the cheese, bringing in the cheese, we shall come rejoicing, bringing in the cheese."

I continued playing possum. They were ready to have this small choir conclude. David was not. Next he sang, "Bringing in the apples." Since he could sing verses of this song for just about all the fruits and vegetables in the garden, I wondered how they were going to get David turned off now that they had him turned on.

While David started singing "Bringing in the potatoes," I recalled a tactic I had learned in a class I had taken. Asking for an offering will act as a stabilizer and bring people who are over-emotional, or out of control, back to normal again. These young people were on their toes. They knew the tactic, too. When David finished "Bringing in the string beans," they asked if he would like to make a donation. I was surprised when he gave them a dollar, as he had never been a generous contributor to religious causes. I was so happy to leave that I forgot to thank them for the hotel list.

We spent two years trying to teach David to ride a bike again. With a new plan, the last try worked. We wheeled the bike out of the bike shop (a girls bike by this time) and David perched himself on the seat. The shop owner slipped David's bad foot in a device that would hold the foot in place on the peddle and gave him a shove. Away David sailed, yelling at the top of his voice, "Hurray! Hurray! I'm riding a bike, Jan! I'm riding a bike! Look at me!" I jumped up and down with joy. I wanted to shout, "Be careful David." But I knew at this time my warning was inappropriate. David was mobile on his own. What impressed me the most was that instead of going diagonally across the street, as he had done before, David went down to the corner, stopped his bike, waited for the traffic and went across the corner appropriately.

It was misty that day, and I was worried that he might not see the cars. Sensing my concern he said, "Don't worry about me, Jan. I'll stay on the sidewalk." And then he was out of sight, in the mist. It was a short block so I could here him yelling all the way, "I am still riding it, Jan! I'm still on the bike! I didn't fall off! I'm still going!" Around the block he came.

I turned to the shop owner and said, "He's riding a bike. Do you understand what that means? He's riding a bike!" The owner looked at me confused. I said, "Please understand it's been five years since he's been able to ride a bike."

Only then did the owner realize that David was ably challenged. David had changed so much that his behavior had not given the owner one clue that he was ably challenged to any extent. Then the owner compassionately said that as a young boy he had a brain injury, and it had taken him two years to recover. So he joined in our triumph. As David whirled back into the yard he said, "I must tell dad. I want to call him. I want to tell him!" Into the bike shop he went.

I can hear him on the phone now, "Dad, dad, I'm riding a bike!" Then I lost all control. Joy overwhelmed me, and words that I had not been able to express through the whole, long ordeal seemed to fill my mind. I found myself sinking to my knees against the wall of the bike shop, in the parking lot with the cars whizzing by, in the now soft rain, letting the cleansing water splash on my face, mingling with my tears I said, "Thank you, Jesus. With all my heart, thank you!" Over and over I kept saying, "Thank you, Jesus!" Why wouldn't these words come before, I wondered? Had I really been bitter without being aware of it? I don't think so. We had just stayed the course, not looking back, going over hurdle after hurdle. Then finally, in that moment David rode the bike, I discovered the rewards for a good fight. I recognized that my Lord had helped me through it all.

ADHD HUNTER

Many times in my life, I believed people viewed my intent, motive, and actions as flawed. In answer to this, when I wasn't a practicing Christian I believed my motives, intent, and actions were wrong. But in later years, when I made a renewal with Christ, one thing I really wanted to understand was why people accused me of certain behaviors and motives that I didn't sense inside my mind and sometimes didn't even understand their point of view. This haunted me into my late years. I went to a psychologist and was tested for Attention Deficit Hyperactivity Disorder. The test proved positive. Knowing that I had ADHD helped me to understand other family members who exemplified some of my characteristics.

In jest, Bill calls it "janooting" because it's a little off from my name Janette. An example of "Janooting:" While at the grocery store I went to the checkout lane to pay for the groceries and realized I left my purse in the car where Bill was waiting. I left my groceries in the cart carrel inside the store and went out to get my purse. I came back in and paid for my groceries then made sure I had my purse. Bill sat quietly in the car reading the newspaper, watching. When I sat down in the car, Bill asked, "Did you forget anything?" I said, "No." He asked the question again, and again I said no. "What are we having for dinner tonight?" he inquired. Then I realized I forgot the groceries. I went back, showed my receipt, retrieved my groceries, and returned to the car where Bill jovially said, "I'm sure glad you got that all figured out!" I hope this section will help us all understand ADHD individuals.

Individuals with Attention Deficit Disorder are referred to by some authors as hunters rather than planters. We are great researchers, police officers, private investigators, authors, and historians. However, like David Warrington, my disorder, ADHD makes it difficult to function each day with any kind of balance. For instance: being able to accept the deferral of personal rewards for doing large amounts of work. This is illustrated by the following activity conducted with children noted in the book, *The Edison Trait*. When the children were told they would receive a small toy immediately for completing a small number of arithmetic problems, each group completed the same number of problems. Then the children were given a choice. They could get a small toy for doing a small amount of work, or they could do a larger amount of work for a much larger toy, but they would not get the bigger toy until two days later. Under these conditions, more of the children with ADHD chose the small, immediate reward for little work. However, the other children were more likely to choose the larger, deferred reward for more work.

In an age when automation has permeated many aspects of society, some become "successful non-conformists." What David deBronkart first wrote about in *The Edison Trait* in 1992, Lucy de Palladino expanded upon again in 1997.[2] She ascribed a genetic susceptibility (50% of occurrences) to ADHD. Cognitive science describes divergent and convergent thinking. Divergent thinking is described as spontaneous, nonlinear brainstorming. Convergent thinking is characterized by linear, logical, sequential reasoning. Learning to keep the balance is the key.

ADHD Individuals will find this a struggle and will appear insecure trying. Yet, it is the trying that challenges us.

While the inventor, Thomas Edison, was unsuccessful in his early school environment and was suspended from school twice by the time he was eight years old, he was later home schooled by his mother. When he left home to work for the rail roads, within months, he invented a timing and signaling device used for nearly a century. His later invention of the light bulb led to a host of other inventions such as the microphone and the motion picture. A similar illustration is that of a young girl whose middle school math teacher said she was "slow" and needed remedial training. With the positive encouragement and push of her father, she began getting tutorial help from a retired math professor and others who taught, not from the "deficiency" perspective but to become *better*. Today, the young lady is an award-winning teacher and is working on her doctorate in math. Both examples illustrate the positive effect of encouragement on humans. Yet, ADHD individuals are often marked non-cooperative when we believe we are being cooperative. I did this when I tried to solve my own problem by finding a quiet place to sew without distraction while in a childhood sewing class.

Teachers laughed at what appeared to be absurdities regarding my needing a quiet place to work because noise distracted my studies. This is now known as standard needs for ADHD affected individuals. In that case, what was thought to be right was no longer accepted as more knowledge about the ably challenged developed. When we believe in an individual, the person is motivated to try and sometimes reaches significant accomplishments through necessity. Increased achievement in youth can be maximized. Even adults who find older mentors are better able to cope. We found mentors from outside the family are often more successful with us because they are able to fulfill the role of friendship when they understand our problems.

Our journey at home with David reflected this kind of coaching. We delighted when he made improvements, even though he did not become independent as we had hoped and the improvements were not always permanent. Set backs have been experienced by both of us. In my case, setbacks have been around all my life. But the hunt, the chase for new tries for success pays off.

I am a Christian hunting the Bible for new truths to better understand God, myself, and others. I have found meadows in my soul in which to rest in Christ. My goals are to point others to the meadows within them where God speaks among the blossoms fragranced with the sweetness of Jesus. This assignment of twenty-seven years as a caregiver for David has systematically challenged me, and others, in the tasks of daily life. For me, challenges to my health have periodically interrupted the course of this book, yet they have been part of my story. Challenges have crossed my path as well as the paths of others as we make the journey, individually and together, with God Almighty paving the way.

ADHD is a relatively new descriptive term for a problem that has gone under many previous names: hyperactivity, minimal brain dysfunction, cerebral dysfunction. The diagnosis "attention deficit disorder" better describes the basis problem – difficulty with concentration and attention span.

As a result of these problems, the Attention Deficit Disorder child senses anger and rejection from others but they cannot seem to understand why. Incredible frustration follows, frequently accompanied by clowning behaviors and tumbling self-esteem. A careful diagnosis is imperative.

Again, we can well see, caregivers are not always chosen, but drafted from all walks of life. Whether they have ADHD or not, they lend a helping hand. It's not always appreciated, but their hands and hearts are open.

ADHD and Caregiver Help

Attention deficit disorder comes in two varieties: ADD with hyperactivity and ADD without hyperactivity. Both varieties have these characteristics in common:

1. *Poor Attention Span.* The child does not finish tasks or work, cannot concentrate or stick with activities or stay on a task.
2. *Distractibility.* The child daydreams and is distracted by even the slightest noises, even his or her own thoughts. The central nervous system normally filters out distractions so people can concentrate on the task at hand. Children with attention deficit disorder have trouble doing this.
3. *Impulsivity.* The child consistently acts without thinking (even though the child knows right from wrong and knows the consequence of misbehavior), shifts one activity to another, frequently blurts out in class, has trouble awaiting his or her turn, and has trouble delaying gratification.

Poor social sense. ADD children tend to miss or misread the nonverbal cues necessary to monitor one's own behavior and tend to say to say and do the wrong things at the wrong time.

❦ 11 ❧

Growing Up in Christ

E MOTIONAL TRAUMA CAN change us. Trying to uproot deep-seated debilitating emotional habits can be traumatic. It's a lot like an adorable completely cared for baby who all of a sudden has to become responsible for their personal habits and behaviors starting with potty training.

When one begins to move away from the newborn Christian stage and into having to be more careful about the responses and reactions, it can be a bit jarring.

No Christian is born of God in complete maturity. Scripture bears this out. In his letter to the Corinthians, Paul said "And I, brethren, could not speak unto you as unto spiritual, but as unto carnal, even as unto babes." "…pulling down strong holds, casting down arguments and every high thing that exalts itself against the knowledge of God, and bringing every thought into captivity. Meaning anger, hate, jealously, and strife. (Corinthians 10:4-6) … But I fear lest somehow as the serpent beguiled Eve…, so your minds should not be corrupted from the simplicity that is in Christ. (Corinthians 11:3)

Carnal thinking and behavior is tolerated more gently in the Lord's dealings with babes in Christ but is less tolerated in long-term Christians because we are held responsible for what we know and for what we have been given.

DIAPER RASH

Why do I say *diaper rash*? When I was going through the process of having God take His surgical knife and dig up the wounds of my past,

I felt a lot of emotional pain. I like to call these fresh wounds "diaper rash." I say diaper rash, first because my pastor often uses that phrase and second because I think it makes it a bit easier to go through the process when we look at it that way. There are two stages of diaper rash. Both stages involve the emotional and spiritual processes of healing anger, hatred, jealousy, envy, strife, and fear—in Biblical terms we would call these the deeds (or toxins) of the flesh.

The first kind of diaper rash is the wounds from the Lord's surgical knife and soreness around the cut where the toxins are released. The embedded soreness that was the hardest for me to overcome occurred when testing proved I had dyslexia and ADHD as well as obsessive compulsive symptoms under stress. Some of my siblings and I were taunted as children about my mother's being in an asylum. Sad to say, there are still some who are insensitive and do not know the circumstances unrelated to my mother's illness. I have learned to accept my diagnosis and profit from it. I've been expected to perform and I have. If we give the waste, or emotional baggage, to the Lord rather than continuing to walk around with the tell-tale signs of the toxins being "smelled" by everyone, the wounds from having the waste come to the surface will heal very quickly. This is especially true if we bathe them in the fresh water of the Word of God and allow God to rub His healing agent, the oil of the Holy Spirit, on them as we bask in His presence.

The secondary kind stage of diaper rash will set in if we keep carrying the load. These will be compounded irritants from "getting rubbed the wrong way" because we are out of sorts due to pain of our primary stage of diaper rash that is not healing. As long as we continue carrying our waste around rather than giving it back to the Lord, we will be irritable and suffer pain. Often, when we will be short with others, impatient, whiney, self-centered, in pain, and just generally uncomfortable no matter what activity we are engaged it.

Oftentimes, we will continue to carry around our waste because of old habits like trying to do it our own way, the bottom line being rebellion in one form or another. When God was taking the surgical knife to me, digging out the "tumors" of the past, forcing me to look at them, and forgiving everyone involved, I often felt emotionally raw. I also felt naked before God because I no longer had "the blankees" of denial to cover up my pain.

Then, early one morning I surrendered all to God; I dumped my dirt and anger that surfaced at the moment on God. He became the Lord of my life and I began learning how to grow into Christ-like behaviors. Through faith, I began placing my damaged emotions, one by one, under the control of God.

Each victory over diaper rash has been glorious to me, because I know I'm shedding more of what has been keeping me from being more Christlike. As I move from one level of learning to another, I seem to go through the same process of discarding babes-in-Christ bad habits and having a pity party at each stage. When I fail, I get up and try again.

There is life beyond opening and closing wounds, however. I call this the "potty training" stage because this is where we begin to exercise restraint. We cannot be used of God unless our natural behavior is changed to a Spirit-controlled behavior that exhibits flexibility, patience, and congeniality with enough creativity to thrive as team players among others with good behaviors. This was true for Paul and it is also true for us. Paul was a hater and murderer of early Christians. He was so persistent he could be referred to as stiff necked (not pliable). He needed to be broken and molded into the Body of Christ to be part of the rich early church harvest for the Lord.

POTTY TRAINING

Some characteristics of those who move through the potty training phase: not ashamed of Christ, good deeds, love, honest, embracing God, grieving for others pain, devoted. Giving, tender, peculiar, encouragers, assisters, poor in spirit, cherished by God, understands others, admired by God, happy, pressing toward a higher calling, and show desire for deeper relationship with God.

Potty training is difficult for some children. To me, being an adult who is being potty trained in Christ is humbling. However, I do know this is necessary because when it is accomplished He chooses us for service.

Sometimes God asks me to do things that seem impossible. I thank God anyway because it strengthens my faith. As we move on through the process of trusting God to the point of doing things that don't make sense to our natural minds, more and more we are leaning on Him and can be used by Him in greater degrees. Tasks that require a greater degree of trust in Him seem less overwhelming because as we move on, the fragrance of our victories in Christ linger, pulling us closer to the sweetness of Jesus. I have Christ to guide me and through His power I can do all things. (Philippians 4:12)

God asking His people to do some things that do not make sense to them is not new. One biblical example of this may be found in the case of Naaman, who felt insulted because he had to wash himself in the dirty Jordan River for God to heal his leprous spots. At first he would not go because the prophet did not come, but sent someone else with the message of the requirement for him to wash himself in the Jordan River.

> So Naaman went down and dipped himself in the Jordan seven times as the man of God had told him, and his flesh was restored and became clean like that of a young boy.
>
> —2 KINGS 5:14

Control over our tongue is an important of reflection of our maturity in Christ, or lack thereof. The Bible tells us that we have rule over our tongue, we have rule over our whole body. God tells me not to gush, but to sprinkle, my enthusiasm without babbling. For example, when I get my attitude right, such as asking forgiveness of my enemy, I want to shout from the hills, "I got it right! Praise God!" Shouting my success to the housetops, however, may breach confidentiality or give the appearance that I am being boastful.

To me, "potty training" is also learning good habits by releasing old or bad habits that plague us and interrupt healthy thinking processes. Mourning prayers under God's direction can bring closure to unnecessary guilt. Offending others may occur when we are angry over change, and when we try to earn our way to heaven. It is a result of not accepting God's delegated authority and their criticism. We can mourn our guilt and give it to Jesus. We can mourn our rudeness.

We can also go through a type of mourning when we forgive people who have been rude to us in the present or even injured us in the past. God's servants of old used sack clothes to show mourning needs. Mourning can wash away pain.

Some people in the Bible mourned when they confessed their wrongdoing. We can also mourn with others as they express their pain, sorrow, sin, and regrets. Jesus can apply healing oil of peace and contentment. Then we leave our cares at Jesus' feet and start afresh. Jesus said, "Therefore if the Son makes you free you shall be free indeed!" (John 8: 36)

Through suffering, humility and brokenness in Christ I'm learning obedience. Some who are not sensitive to sin do not connect obedience to God with obedience to God's delegated authority.

This type of self-restraint is seen in our responses to delegated authority in the home, the church, workplace, and community. In the home, for instance, Christ delegates the authority to the husband. A wife under her husband's authority obeys him, but first she obeys God, which may be different. I need to understand my spouse's abilities, wants, and needs. I cannot be selfish and say "I am doing this for God" when I am doing things at the expense of my spouse's peace of mind. God does not honor what causes friction or unhappiness in our home unless the Spirit is trying to show us there is a need for change. A marriage that is ordered by the Lord, and therefore a happy one, will be full of restraint because the husband and wife will be serving one another in love and in the fear of the Lord. We will not be dumping our concerns on one another at the drop of every hat, but will restrain ourselves until a time when our spouse is ready to hear what we have to say—or when it is clearly the timing of the Lord.

In my case, however, I have good intentions but again I am disorganized. I start two or three parts of an assignment at once, sometimes doing the middle part first. When a leader wants an update, or others are complaining they cannot follow my thinking process, all concerned can become perplexed. When I tell him/her how I have been doing the assignment, the look on his/her face could be much like the grandmother's in the following story.

There was a little girl who wanted to help her sick grandmother so she made a cup of tea. She first boiled the water then poured it through a strainer where there were tea leaves in place to insure taste. The grandmother was impressed until the little girl said, "I couldn't find a tea strainer so I used the fly swatter, but don't worry I didn't use the new one."

As I have learned to walk under the restraint of God's will by obeying Him, my joy in Him as grown fuller and fuller. Obeying Him rather than going back to my old ways of coping, especially during difficult times, has been much easier when I have kept in mind that God has a good plan for my life and His ways are higher than mine. Along with this, the more attune I am to His voice because of my intimate relationship with Jesus Christ, the more peace and contentment I have. Taking my burdens to Him and leaving them there adds up to living in the New Testament Sabbath of resting in Him always, of resting from our own labors and taking His easy yoke, His will, upon me. Sure, I can interrupt His plan at any time by not listening to His counsel, and so with that in mind, I am careful to never again put my relationship with Him on the back burner.

NEW BEHAVIORS

Characteristics of some of those who move up through the "potty training" stage are as follows: Insightful into God's word, genuine, thankful, fair, virtuous, calm, covered by the blood, truthful, willing, invited, welcomed, pleased, humble, nursing, healed, elevate others, forgiving, just, preserved, good conduct, ready, wonderful, charming in Christ, clean mind, spirit led, gentle, convinced of God, broken, comforters, without murmur, good mannered, joyful, faithful, hope, fragrance of Christ, obedient, embraced by followers of Christ, yielded to accept God's delegated authority, does warfare against Satan, sensitive without argue, new each morning, returned to Christ.

Dave Williams, author of *Growing Up God's Way*, describes very well the stages of growing up in Christ. [1]

Baby Traits

1. We have jealousy. Why are his/her ideas accepted when mine make more sense?
2. Why does the pastor listen to him/her when I have been a part of the church for years and know much more about what's going on and what should or should not be?
3. The pastor never talks to me. Many of us feel this way sometimes.

A newborn babe was left by the side of the road by his mother and was soon covered with ant bites and other insects. Near death, the baby was taken to the hospital by a passerby who heard his cry. When we leave those who are hurting without help, we could cause spiritual death.

Children

1. Children talk, talk, talk. A baby becomes a child when the non-stop talking begins.
2. Children try to make an impression. They say, "Watch me. I can do this when I'm only three years a Christian, when others who have been in "The Way" longer are spiritually dying."
3. Also, we are very cliquey at this stage and do not reach out beyond our circle. We are like Peter and John on the Mount of Transfiguration. We are so glorified in one spot, with one group, that we forget we are here to win the lost.

Children and adolescents form cliques. The difference between a clique and a group of friends or participants in something is this: Those who form cliques can make a statement with body language, excuses, or bluntly stating, "You're not one of us." A healthy group may meet together at certain times or places but do not discourage others who might want to join unless there is a valid reason, such as, "Tickets are sold out."

Adolescents in Christ are very easily offended. Instead, some think, "I have a right to be offended." I have read many books on the offended and, generally speaking, I believe, along with others, that the easily offended are often those who are unhappy in daily living. They hope to feel lifted by volunteer efforts.

Adulthood Stage

Here are some signs of spiritual maturity:

- More implicit and universal trust in God.
- A separation from the world and an increasing deadness to all the world has to offer.
- Less temptation to sins of omission (example: neglect of prayer, Bible reading, etc.).
- A growing steadiness and intensity of zeal in promoting the cause of Christ.
- Less *self*-consciousness and more *Jesus*-consciousness.
- A growing deadness to the praise of men.
- A growing warmth and sincere acceptance of the whole will of God.
- A growing calmness and quietness under great afflictions.
- A growing patience under much provocation.
- Joyfulness even when disappointments come.
- Less temptation to gripe, complain, criticize, and murmur.
- Less temptation to resentment and the attitude of retaliation when insulted, criticized, or abused.
- Less temptation to dwell upon and magnify our trials and troubles.
- Less anxiety about the future.
- Less inclination to speak uncharitably about another individual.
- A growing readiness to forgive others and forget old injuries.
- An increasing naturalness in treating people kindly and praying for them.
- Finding it easier and easier to make wholehearted sacrifices.
- We find ourselves more and more impressed with revelations of Bible truths.
- A growing jealousy for the honor of God, and for the honor and purity of His Church.[2] The New Life...You can get off to a great start on your exciting life with Jesus! Prepare for something wonderful.

❦ 12 ❦

Receiving Help From the Church

HAD LIFE BEEN so full of trials, doubts, agonies, and perplexities that I must wither and moan as a caregiver rather than persevere to know all God has for me? At the beginning of this calling to care I was no warmer than an unmovable lukewarm Christian. I did not let disturbances penetrate deep enough to know I was dead in the Spirit. I did not know the triumph of becoming alive in my soul again.

The sorrow, hurt, and grief that left me empty was my motivation to do something to move forward. To be a burned-out caregiver is something I am acquainted with. The question was, "Could I make a recovery?" Trying to do so without Christ could make me obnoxious, timid, and afraid, using a clamor of words as my cover. I could fall and get up again and again. I wondered what approach would break the bondage that makes me quiver and turn to stronger personalities for support or to help my pain. but I feel troubled if controlled. I push others away.

I prayed to God, "Burned-out and with troubles I can still find You stirring in my soul. Thank you, Jesus, thank you!"

WAYS LEADERS MAY CREATE A SAFE CHURCH ENVIRONMENT FOR CAREGIVERS

Government services are not a substitute for the integration of faith and service in the church. Some government leaders at the highest level, including U.S. President George Bush, are in fact working to give faith-based initiatives funding support.

What caregivers and providers need is a place of rest in the Lord. The Old Testament's rigid Sabbath law provided a structured time to make whole again by approaching the Throne of Grace for timely help; a sacred pause in the ordinary labor of earning bread.[1] The New Testament extends the spirit of the law to include common sense, such as Jesus picking corn on the Sabbath for something to eat. This was a new dawn, the spirit of rest, transcending and fulfilling the reason for the law. The church may serve in helping caregivers take better care of their own spiritual well-being in preparation for immortal life in Heaven.

Certainly, Dr. Harold Shindoll's, founder of the University of Florida Christian University, book *Grace and Sovereignty of God* is effective in bringing this to our attention. "A proper release on Him provides the balance we need to find rest and peace in our daily lives." [1]

A Call to Change

I have had wonderful pastors who have helped me so much in making a "comeback," and I am a grateful Christian. Legalism is difficult for me, partly because I have an attention span deficit. Brad Watson's excellent book, *Is it Lust or Legalism* can point to something we all may need to consider when we have rules we feel work so well they cannot be changed.[2] In the conclusion of his book he states, "Maybe it's time for an update." I also think legalism can be particularly damaging to the burned out caregiver because Jesus Christ fulfilled the Mosaic Law and if we try to go back to nit picking over dos and don't's but miss the larger issues, the hurting will not know they are free to live the life of peace and rest for which Jesus lived, died, on rose again.

Healing on the Sabbath

> And it came to pass also on another Sabbath, that he entered into the synagogue and taught; and there was a man whose right hand was withered.

> And the scribes and Pharisees watched him, whether he would heal on the Sabbath day; that they might make accusations against him.
>
> But he knew their thoughts and said to the man which had the withered hand, Rise up, and stand forth, and he arose and stood forth.
>
> Then he said Jesus unto them, I ask you one thing; Is it lawful on the Sabbath day to do good, or to do evil? To save life, or to destroy it?
>
> And looking round about upon them all, he said unto them, Stretch forth thy hand. And he did so: and his hand was restored whole as the other.
>
> —LUKE 6–10

When I sat under traditional non-updated messages I felt I needed to bark like a dog over and over, calling attention to the saga of unmet caregiving needs. Some may need a different brand of food. I could not find a place to air my needs and suggestions for more emotional, spiritual and grief-support; a place such as a healing center or a ministry of trained men and women when I was desperate.

LEADERS NEED TO RESPOND IN NEW WAYS

God uses pastors who use God's power to lead. They have resources available to them that laymen may not necessarily have. I have not known a pastor yet who when asked would not share a point or two along the way regarding available needed resources for spiritual healing. I believe all denominations are doing a good job but, in general, developing more healing centers or healing teams can help. Caregivers can benefit from such expertise.

Carry each other's burdens and in this way you will fulfill the law of Christ. If anyone thinks he is something when he is nothing, he deceives himself. Each one should test their own actions. Then he can take pride in himself, without comparing himself to somebody else, for each one should carry his own load.

The noted John Maxwell, in one of his conferences, indicated that a church leader is a true caregiver when he can look at his churches congregation and see God's empowered stars who can move and shake others into action. Instead of inhibiting these people with so much structure they cannot experiment, catch their coat tails and move up with them as God leads them into areas of visionary growth. Without discouragement, they will shed errors as they move along with the Spirit.

MINISTER IN A WAY THAT INVITES THE WORK OF THE HOLY SPIRIT

During a time when I was struggling with being burned out from my work as being a caregiver to David and with being ably challenged with ADHD and bouts of Obsessive Compulsive Disorder when under stress, the Lord led us to a wonderful church where our warmhearted pastor had a reputation for delivering sermons with fire and heart-felt eloquence. I believed he had true charity from God. He lifted Bill's and my hearts in earnest prayer to God and expressed the Lord's goodness in a world of thorns, temptations, troubles, and cares. For the first time, I felt like caregiving the ably challenged (me) was a cure for my shallow soul. He presented such sweet morsels of excellence in Christian living, I was sure his worship services were a forerunner of Heaven.

HOLD UP A STANDARD FOR RIGHTEOUSNESS

Like with anyone else, it is important for people struggling with the needs of caring for or being an ably challenged to be held accountable for godly standards of right and wrong. In summation, sin must be called sin. An example of what happens when people are fed intoxicating messages rather than the pure Word of God may be seen in an epiphany I had while my husband and I were on vacation one summer, I sat at a sidewalk café while Bill toured a historic site. The tour company we were using provided champagne as hospitality for the busload of tourists at this particular site. There were many half-full champagne glasses left on the café tables by the tourists.

I was enjoying my tea when I noticed how strange the pigeons were acting. I am not afraid of pigeons if they are acting like pigeons, but these pigeons were flopping all over the place and walking sideways.

One tipped over onto my shoe and then looked up at me as if to say, "I'm still a pigeon, although I'm not acting like one." These pigeons had been flying onto the tables and drinking the leftover champagne.

Looking back on those drunken pigeons reminds me of Christians who state they are Christians living in sin but do not walk a straight line with Christ. Being blinded by our limitations and failing to recognize God's power can lead to this kind of compromise.

Holding up the standard for righteousness, however, extends to into the community as well because the church as a whole has a responsibility of being bearers of the Good News and the banner of the Lord out side the church walls. Helping caregivers look beyond their own circumstances, and to caring for the fields of harvest, is a way of strengthening their Christian resolve to fight the good fight of faith for a purpose that is even larger than themselves or their own families.

> To me, those we see in church are not the only ones who need help. The church must campaign for decency and morality with elevated standards. It sets the moral tone for all through preaching, exhorting, counseling, or God-directed protesting, addressing poor conduct. The church should lead in Christian ministries, teachings, practices for fellowship, and meaningful living. The love, prayers, and salvation that the church sets in motion are our guide for Christian living and hope for now and all times. This is my hope.
>
> —Author unknown

I believe that churches can grow in effectiveness through fervent prayer, clear vision, faith-based goals and priorities, uncluttered teachings and delegation throughout the anointed body. A warm exciting atmosphere will foster healing, worship, discipleship, and evangelism.

Trained to Recognize the Scope of Caregivers' Needs

Loving servants can accept the job of caregiving because they have the gift of mercy. They are the ones who, by their very spiritual gift, are helpers and alleviators of pain and suffering. But we must accept the fact that we cannot be all things to the ones who need us. We learned this first hand. As caregivers, we need to be on guard. Caregivers must be firmly grounded in biblical truths. We are not immune to feelings of frustration and just plain exhaustion particularly when drafted. Caregiving can be a 24-hour-a-day job.

When laymen who have not been trained and do not have God's anointing try to provide guidance, it is very likely that their advice will need support from Christian experts to divert from dire consequences. However, some well-meaning pastors who are not sensitive to the real needs of caregivers may minimize their needs and thereby heap added guilt on them that may lead them to leave the church setting altogether. In our case, two separate pastors did not know the scope of pain present in two separate caregivers. They responded similarly by emphasizing that they get tired also, and that could be true.

To us, it sounded like these pastors needed a break. Again, where needed, why not develop a church healing center to accommodate those who demonstrate this need? We have family camp and children's camp, why not a healing center? Influence at healing centers can help our sad or debilitated brothers and sisters in Christ. If caught in time, before bitterness sets in, we believe this thinking can be turned around fairly quickly so they can move forward. I remembered that Jesus walked away from John the Baptist when he was despairing in prison. Jesus could have saved his cousin but this was not the purpose for which He came. Sometimes, learning to walk away from what we cannot change is our answer—burned out caregivers have to at times. Counseling can help. John the Baptist fulfilled his purpose, as painful as it was.

Helping in Practical Ways

We love all who teach or share the Word of God to caregivers who are seeking ways to prevent burnout. God can help others see that life is worth living at many levels of function. God can use willing people. There are practical ways in which the church can be a source of strength to all concerned. One church sends food and babysitters to help with children and the homebound adults in times of tragedy or trauma. Thus, caregivers who do not always sense they are burning out can be just as wounded as the man helped by the Good Samaritan. The Good Samaritan, being the caregiver in this situation, gave assistance that helped the man to heal and begin to cope with the physical situation in which he found himself.

> But a certain Samaritan traveling that way came to him. And seeing him, he was moved with pity. And coming near, he tied up his wounds, pouring on oil and wine. And putting him on his own animal, he brought him to an inn and tool care of him. And on the next day, going away, he took out two coins and gave them to the innkeeper. And said to him, take care of him, and whatever you may spend that is more than this, I will repay you when I come back.
>
> —LUKE 10:33–35

Some churches provide a setting for a common meal on a regular basis, thus recognizing and supporting the special needs of the families with an opportunity to network. Families who have loved ones who are ably challenged can engage in mutual support and give practical suggestions on issues they are currently facing or have already dealt with.

Systems at the Rehabilitation Institute of Michigan found that social support improved the caregiver's sense of well-being, helped the injured to recover, and indicated the caregiver becoming depressed can interrupt cognitive behavioral post-injury problems. Considering these findings, I believe depression in the traumatized and the caregiver seems to hinder progress for all involved.

I believe that through Christ we can learn to point the needy one to counseling, spiritual support, and understanding. Unlike Marie Antoinette, who exposed her insensitivity to the real issue of no bread by replying to the starving people of France, "Let them eat cake," our replies can reach the life of the Church in our quest for greater heights.

Author and Christian counselor, Larry Crabb, indicates in his wonderful book, *Connecting,* that in some cases, a trained lay person helps.[3] Yet another author cautioned that we should be careful, because a religion junkie can come on "smooth" but may be controlling. Church members are not trained psychologists and yet they are often asked to understand people as they unload their sin and try to get their lives straightened out.

Some ask, "What do families with ably challenged members who are not church members need?" I believe all families have some basic need for respite. Churches differ in circumstances and resources. What is available will vary. Forming a consortium of churches where resources can be pooled together for small rural, urban, or suburban churches has been done. The commonality is in that these families need God.

We may, as Christian educators, want to look again at whom we receive and do not receive for full educational credits from other Christian schools or learning institutions that have similar gospel teachings if proofs of doctrine are acceptable. Dare we "split hairs" when it comes to the ably challenged being qualified to go forward and serve their calling for Christ? To me, it's futuristic when our Christian institutions have a track for full credit higher education that serves the ably challenged, and many do. I believe students should meet the expectations of the track. However, if the learning institution does not have full credit tracks or it's not possible to get with the ably challenged and adopt alternatives, should we be slow to accept transfer credits?

In some family settings where the caregiving task has been taken up by the only willing member and others are not willing to participate, particularly where there are ailing parents or ably challenged siblings, unfair remarks come under the guise of "we're behind you and when you can no longer do this, we'll support you in whatever decision you have to make." In my experience, the loving servant not only has the burden of the care, but also the guilt when the hard decisions come.

Centers could help caregivers deal with guilt. The caregiver cannot make others see the light or responsibility when they refuse. It can be heartbreaking. The caregiver needs Jesus' healing touch. The decision of putting the loved one in a different living situation out of the home is tough on those left with the responsibility. Caregivers need help in recognizing when it is time to let go before it causes greater unhappiness and discomfort for the loved one. Can we, as the body of Christ, show caregivers God's healing ways?

Even though Bill and I had much support from our children, we would need added support from our church and pastor in the spring of 2002 when David's weight fell to 125 against his height of 5'9". He leaned over when he sat. He ate little and was literally wasting away before our eyes. An appointment was made with his first-rate neurologist in Warren, Michigan.

It was recommended that he become a resident in a facility for the brain injured in the Detroit area temporarily where he would have easy access to medical testing facilities.

David spent the summer there while several tests cleared up the questions about the weight loss. It was a combination of factors both mental and physical. It was then recommended he be placed in a wonderful residence for brain injured in our city. We thought we could not part with David after twenty-seven years. Our kids insisted. We could no longer keep up the pace to insure the future. Our heart broke in two.

Our response was not a unique one: social worker Holly Fortin Smith indicated to a Detroit talk show host, Cynthia Conty, that in many cases when long-term caregivers of family members make the decision to place the loved one they care for into an assisted living facility (could include loved one's death), the caregiver may emotionally "crash." This happened in our situation. Talk therapy flowed out of my mouth involuntarily. Whoever was closest heard my reactions. Bill handled things differently. When he is worn out he simply sleeps.

BE AFFIRMING BUT MINDFUL OF THE POSSIBILITY OF LARGER ISSUES

It is important for pastors and lay leaders to know the difference between self-esteem and self-respect. Self-esteem is recognizing one's own gifts and talents that are to be developed and used. Self-respect is using these talents without tactics like manipulating, tattling, whispering, emotional blackmail, or other inter-self defeating tactics.

Some may be floundering because they do not feel they are being affirmed and are therefore using unstable or forceful unhealthy behavior to find help for their needs. Some may have had other negative church experiences and are transferring their reactions to the pain in those old circumstances into their present church life. Others may have seemingly impossible home or personal situations with no easy solutions. In these instances, more formal counseling may be advised, especially if they have been prone to move from church to church and will probably not receive the needed help if the pastor or leader does not intervene quickly.

However rationally intended, there are times when behavior and information can seem odd, even to ourselves.

GUARD THEM FROM SPIRITUAL PREDATORS

Caregivers are so mentally tired they do not probe for those who would bring them false doctrine. A caregiver can be approached by counterfeit religion just by opening their front door to someone carrying a Bible, but who also is carrying messages from a cult. One way to help the caregiver, whether church member or not, is to fill the voids before the enemy of their souls attempts to do it in some other way.

> Beware of the false prophets, who come to you in sheep's clothing, but inwardly are ravenous wolves.
>
> —MATTHEW 7:15, NAS

GUARD THEM FROM EMOTIONAL PREDATORS

Church leaders and lay people may also help caregivers by lovingly helping them to be on the lookout for emotional blackmail and manipulation that may threaten their emotional stability. Caregivers may encounter these manipulations directly through the person in their care or from people within the church, or they may encounter them indirectly if the person in his/her care becomes the victim of manipulation.

Here is an example: A child who is less mature can sometimes go to extremes to win a more mature child's approval. He will then become a slave of the other's. My five-year-old great-grandson runs after older kids trying to join in their play. They are rude to him when he joins with lesser-developed play skills. Sometimes they take advantage of him, getting him to run after a wild ball pitched in softball or to get them drinks. Then they hide from him. Another example: Youth, in their eagerness for God, can unknowingly feel justified in making the elderly seem less than capable.

Satan uses powerful negative messages on children of dependent adults and seniors who are confined. "I've been damaged because you were not there for me yesterday," or refusing to eat or talk, or becoming sick when the caregiver makes plans to be away from their charge are examples. There can be threats such as "I'll run away if you go and leave me" and remarks such as "I wouldn't go away and leave someone I cared about," as a ploy. Yet as hard as it is not to walk away from what we believe is manipulation there is always the chance there is an honest need or reasonable explanation. The caregiver needs to stay transparent and have an advocate's attitude toward the challenged one so as not to be drawn into wrong assumptions, talk down, exaggerate reactions, or judge without proof. This can cause stubbornness or breached communications for all concerned. Caregivers often need to regroup from this kind of pressure, and proper respite can become a problem. We may ask ourselves, "What can we, as a body of Christ, do to help?"

Ably challenged persons still need to be held responsible for their behavior. Their peers will sometimes indicate their disapproval verbally or through their actions. Caregivers are counseled to maintain personal boundaries to avoid over-identification and subsequent emotional exhaustion that could be misinterpreted as sin or unknowingly over identifying with a controller.

LEAVE ROOM FOR GROWTH

Compromise may also result when we rely too heavily on other Christians. Although help comes from God through Christian servants, including pastors, we can sometimes be so relieved that we transfer our gratefulness to God's servants and become too attached to them. Our hopes must be in Christ alone. Much heartache may be avoided if our eyes and hearts are fixed on Jesus and not on men.

When under stress, babes-in-Christ or the newly restored can be misunderstood and/or inappropriate under stress. Sometimes our behavior, to others, can seem worse than before restoration as we try to work through problems to get results. We are like Paul, full of zeal.

After his conversion, Paul set out on his own to preach the Gospel without any experience. It is thought, when he went home to Tarsus to try and preach, the believers there were afraid of him because of his conduct before his conversion.

Offer Classes Featuring Guest Speaker

One way to head off problems before they emerge is to prepare congregants on how to be caregivers in advance of the need for them to step into that role in their own lives. The need for training on how to take care of elderly parents is a pretty universal one, particularly now that baby boomers are coming into the retirement setting and problems related to decisions about their care are compounded by the fact that their children have been in multiple marriages. Discussions need to be made as to who will be the primary advocate. The parents should always feel their children are advocates rather than demanding or dictating policies that may not necessarily be in the elderly parent's best interest. Where there are unresolved issues, a concerned professional of elderly caregiving could smooth out problems, issues, and concerns for all involved.

Ways Leaders May Create a Safe Church Environment for the Ably Challenged

A flock of wild geese, which mate for life, graced the sky as they headed for their southern winter home. One pair did not sense a pond was frozen and dropped out of the sky only to land on ice. One bird hit with such force that the ice gave way, breaking both its legs. The ice held fast and froze solid around the bird's legs and would not let it fly. The mate hovered over the bird bringing food and fighting off any foes for an extended length of time. Thanks to the care from the bird's mate, the ice formed a cast around its legs, holding them still. When human hands saw the dilemma, the ice around the bird was broken. The bird came forth from the icy water in perfect condition then the pair flew off together.

Again, I believe church healing teams, along with healing centers, can be more effective with some knowledge of the diagnoses (if possible) of the seeker for proper results. A pharmaceutical company's brochure, left at my general practitioner's office as a public service, reasoned that when life takes an unexpected change you are faced with many psychological situations that call for adjustments, like the bird's situation, in a pattern of outward flowing ripples.

For some people, talk therapy and antidepressant medication is the most effective way to treat depression. Talking with a Christian psychiatrist or another qualified health care professional, which can be offered at a Christian healing center, can help your loved one learn more about depression and other disorders along with the team members, their feelings, how to cope with events that can effect the future. God, the first Healer, along with other healers, can help us learn to cope with events. I recommend Christian professional help when the first steps in prayer have already been used.

In the bird story, human hands were like God assisting. God and human hands relieved my OCD through respite and proper medications. God provides peace and joy to caregivers, along with keeping our health, sanity, and humor intact.

LEARN WHAT YOU CAN ABOUT THE PERSON'S DIAGNOSIS

I believe that a pastor should, if at possible, be made aware of the medical diagnosis of an ably challenged person because, for example, learning that a new convert or church attendant has been diagnosed with ADHD, or other ably challenged disorders, will help the pastor to better understand and be prepared for how this person reacts to situations and may affect others.

Then, the pastor may prepare himself by doing added research on the condition and may learn, for example, that ADHD that is combined with bouts of Obsessive Compulsive Disorder (OCD) behavior can manifest as talking too much to others in person or on the phone. When bouts of OCD are rare, such as at times of grief, individuals showing the behavior can return to normal. The book, *Obsessive Compulsive Disorder: Theory, Research, and Treatment* cites triggers of OCD other than grief.[4]

As we grow older, many of our poor habits which could stem from our genes or even general aging can be harder to hold at bay without miraculous healing from God using a community of doctors. In essence, old individuals may be unable to cope or know how to grasp proper skills to cope. The results can lead to behavioral rituals involving unwilling people or public places in a means of relieving stress. It can be a momentary quick fix; then out of the blue, old appears again from other lack of coping skills. This continues until others force stoppage socially or otherwise not interacting with the inflicted one.

Since many diagnoses can be inherited, including old, if it shows up in other family members, it can be assumed that it is genetic. However, it can occur otherwise. A word of caution: medication that can treat problems should not be ignored in favor of alternatives that haven't provided proven results. ADHD and OCD's symptoms of obsession such as obsessing, hording, pacing, religious obsession, being exact, repetitive rituals, counting compulsion, superstitious and exaggerated fears, lucky and unlucky numbers. Some people can stand up in church and state obscenities or mention voices which suggest harm to others. Anything that is generally different from the loving, caring God who asks us to good needs to be looked into. God can miraculously heal but He may use doctors, counselors who can properly diagnose and/or test with greater benefits and prescribe medication. I recommend these options not be ruled out. The pastor, being prepared with this kind of information, could be crucial to the quality of support which the church might provide for individuals and their families with these disorders.

How the Church May Help Those Diagnosed as Terminally Ill

After initial testing that proves positive, those with terminal illnesses can begin to understand through counseling that he/she is not alone. It's a good opening to share individuals who know they are going to die can still live productive lives within their limits.

Moses, according to the Old Testament, was confined to the desert knowing he would not live to see the Promise Land. He was confined to the desert as God directed his life. Perhaps he helped the children of Israel to look for flowers to lift them up in a dry and thirsty land. The desert can be beautiful with many colors changing day-by-day and season-by-season. God gave Moses the grace to make that final trip to the mountain of Sinai to meet his maker. Moses, Caleb, and Joshua were in tune with God. They could have helped the children of Israel who were under God's judgment of death in the desert rather the Promised Land find short term goals to make as fulfilling as possible. God did not desert his people just as He doesn't abandon the terminally ill now. My first husband, Bob, and I tried to make short-term goals, but it was not always easy.

The apostle Paul continued to preach the nature of Jesus to both the Jews and Gentiles. They began to see Jesus' truth and goodness. Jesus died for everyone, including the terminally ill, and sent the Holy Spirit at Pentecost to help terminally ill believers from then on to have the presence of the Holy Spirit in them to help in difficult times, including death. Help the terminally ill individual understand this whenever possible and make it personal. Those with terminal illnesses will no doubt learn that a great many people will be involved in their lives than he/she never could have possibly anticipated. They can be specialists in insurance, social service agencies in therapy and counseling programs, there are professionals in hospitals, including doctors, nurses and other more intense death awareness teams, peers, friends, family volunteers and acquaintances will also likely be involved either by choice or default. Openness about the reality of their illness is based on each individual's circumstance. Although the terminally ill individual will not feel like a star in this arena, he/she is the focal point.

God does take care of his people when He is in them and they are in Him. He will lead His pastors, churches, and the body of Christ to provide for the needs of His people and for those who are the focus of this book.

The following poem was read aloud in the clubhouse of one of the retirement communities Bill and I lived at. It could apply to any unsung caregiving hero in church.

Someone locks and unlocks the doors.
Someone decorates and undecorates the hall.
Someone organizes shuffling and bowling.
Someone gets doughnuts for our coffee hour.
Someone supervise the food events of our group.
Someone arranges for our garbage to be picked up.
Someone pays our bills.
Someone turns the coffee urns on each Tuesday morning.
Someone plans musical and entertainment activities.
Someone gets our chairs fixed.
The list of someones goes on and on.

Some of these someones are very visible, such as officers, board members, and the coffee committee. Other someones contribute less often and are less visible. Other someones are practically invisible because they contribute but no one sees them. I want to thank all these someones, past, present, and future, who contribute so much to God. And when you get asked to be that someone, say yes, for without you someones, our Church would be in real trouble.

—BILL WARRINGTON

❦ 13 ❧

Learning to Hear the Voice of God in Self-Talk

Sometimes I think my going on and on with "blah, blah, blah," or babbling, makes my conversation seems like an accumulation of leftover, processed words that fix a certain flavor that need not be mentioned out loud. Doesn't the Bible say we should come to Christ like a child? That's how I enjoy coming to the Throne of Grace. I babble to Jesus like a child and He understands all of it where others may wonder.

Could this be Attention Deficit Hyperactivity Disorder, Obsessive Compulsive Disorder, and/or Diaper Rash?

> But God hath chosen the foolish things of the world to confound the wise; and God hath chosen the weak things of the world to confound the things which are mighty.
>
> —1 Corinthians 1:27

On one occasion, we were having a small-group meeting in a new church member's home. We had just moved to our permanent residence in Michigan after living in Huntersville for 17 years. Our house there sold quickly, so the piles of stuff from two houses—one in Huntersville and one from the retirement center in mid-Michigan—did not seem to diminish. Unpretentiously, I asked at prayer time at the small church group if we could pray that God would give me strength to remove or reduce the piles of seemingly worthless items.

The following gives us an idea of how individuals with ADHD like me can react hyperactively in their thinking and problem-solving processes. The mind can run from one thing to another under pressure and thus communicate what others might regard as "babbling."

Each person in the group prayed. I did not have enough faith to believe silent praying for my stack of piles would do the trick so I jumped right in and asked God out loud to reduce the piles. As I prayed, I thought about the other kind of "piles" that an older couple might be inflicted with and in pain. I felt embarrassed and should have shut up right then and there, but my "blah, blah, blah" was on a roll. I had hemorrhoids once myself and it was most unpleasant.

As I continued in prayer, my mind wandered to the fact that I had once had hemorrhoids, which are also sometimes called piles, so I went on praying along that line now, "Please God, note the piles I'm praying about are not hemorrhoids, but piles of stuff to put away, but if any one here has hemorrhoids please help them too."

Then it came to me, maybe someone is suffering and I have insulted him/her by putting their hemorrhoid condition on display. I let out all the stops and prayed, "Oh Lord, you are a God of hemorrhoids too. Place your healing power upon us all."

I often blurt things out and notice astonished looks on faces during my tale telling. At these moments I'm never quite sure what infraction I have violated, but I know that I must have done something.

One night God called me to be a neighborhood church pastor. Does God really speak to our mind? Of course! He communicated to my self-talk. We all talk to ourselves in our mind, but God can and does direct our self-talk when we let Him. It is like someone, something injects a precious fluid into my self-talk. My Holy Spirit directed self-talk is sweet. My God-filled self-talk is so clear. One particular time it helped me sense an angel beside me. "I'm absolutely going crazy," I thought. I was sure an angel was comforting me when I was in pain. "I'm imagining things." I couldn't see the angel, but I knew it was there. I got out of bed and staggered into the living room and opened a Bible to the book of Matthew. I read about Jesus' last supper with his disciples. I read about Jesus dying on the cross. The Holy Spirit spoke to my mind, "I am your Intercessor."

I broke down and sobbed to Jesus Christ. I blurted out all my lifetime pains and hurts since I was a child. I knew God was listening. My main concern was for my husband.

"Jan, will you give your husband to me? I'll take care of him. Will you turn him over to me?" God asked.

I answered, "Oh yes, I'll turn Bill over to you."

Then the self-talk asked, "How about your 'blah, blah, blah?'" "You want my blah, blah, blah?" I answered. "My precious blah, blah, blah that has gotten me through so many trying times. I must have my blah, blah, blah. Oh dear."

I had "blah, blah, blah" for all occasions. It has been my cover for pain throughout my life. Yet, at times it has gotten me into trouble.

My self-talk interrupted my thoughts and asked, "What drives you besides passion, Jan?"

I answered, "Anger and 'blah, blah, blah.' That's what got me through my first book, *The Humpty Dumpty Syndrome.*"

"Don't you think if anger and 'blah, blah, blah' can produce one book, my love could guide you through another?" I believe God, through my self-talk, inquired. "Perhaps so," I thought, "I could try."

"I will guide your 'blah, blah, blah.' Will you turn your anger over to me?" the self-talk continued to inquire.

Although I am glad I gave my 'blah, blah, blah' to Jesus, it was very difficult to let go. I laughed at the idea of trying to give up my 'blah, blah, blah.' I was such an emotional mess. I was sure by then that no one wanted to hear it but Jesus. I longed for an old-fashioned prayer meeting.

"Let's talk again about Sister Lena's class meeting held once a month at your aunt and uncle's county church home when you were a child." (After a Spirit-filled testimony, Sister Lena would often quiz us about our soul. Then she would pray for us and those who were downhearted could go to the altar and pray.)

Then I heard my Jesus say to me, "Writing about your 'blah, blah, blah' is a good place to start."

This is quite a subject. I'm going totally out of my mind. Haven't some people been telling me my 'blah, blah, blah' was boring? Was God really telling me that I had developed and perfected this 'blah, blah, blah?'

My Christ-filled self-talk continued, "You know, Jan, you're not the only one in the world with 'blah, blah, blah' problems. All kinds of things are said about Me.

God said through my self-talk, "My Son, Jesus, carried the burden of the whole world. He died on the Cross for all sinners. Many rejected Me with their 'blah, blah, blah,' but you have come back to Me, and that makes it worth it all."

The people in my family are all great storytellers. We can 'blah, blah, blah' others right out the door. Even if cars are coming in the street, we don't notice because we are so caught up in our talk. A car would have to hit us before we would stop a story. I thought it was in my genes, but I gave up my 'blah, blah, blah' to God and asking Him to help me to be a better listener while at the same time using this characteristic for His purposes. In essence, I gave my 'blah, blah, blah' to His control.

God gave me tongue exercises to remind me my tongue was my worst problem. Sometimes He blasted it with His Spirit, making it tingle to promote awareness and bring my tongue under His control.

> But the natural man receiveth not the things of the Spirit of God: for they are foolishness unto him: neither can he know them, because they are spiritually discerned.
> —ISAIAH 9:6

One night, I woke up and my self-talk voice explained that part of my thinking would be placed back in my subconscious and other thinking would be brought forward. I could have a part in the decision if I so chose. Christ always leaves the final choice up to us. I agreed and then said good night to the part of me that I didn't like. God pushed it into my subconscious. It was the side of me that reacted to situations too quickly with excessive anger, discouragement, moodiness, and enthusiasm. The free-spirited side of me went off picking daisies, without a care in the world, while the practical part of me took the fall when my anger, guilt, and shame rose up in response. I was paying a big price for my nonchalant attitude when really I did care.

The part of me that goes off picking daisies is excessive while the part of me that likes to get things done pays a great price. For instance, when my house is cluttered and I have an unannounced guest who might judge the mess, the protocol conscious part of me is embarrassed and I mentally beat myself up. "Why can't I be more organized?" I ask. Truly, the mind is a battlefield.

"Okay," my God controlled self-talk said, "I am going to bring your 'get-up-and-go' side of you out, and put the 'pick-the-daises' part back in your subconscious."

The other half of me then came out. I had been talking to God for hours and the sun had already started to come up. Where was this all going? The Lord, in my self-talk said, "Jan, I want you to tell Me your heartaches while this side of you is in control." So I did. In essence, I "tattled" on my other half. I told God all of the pains I have had over the years because of enthusiastically started projects, left unfinished when my enthusiasm wore off. I told how my daydreaming got me behind, and caused relationship problems. I was saddened when people didn't appreciate my last minute notices, and yet I had this other side of me that didn't care how long projects took if I liked what I was doing.

As I poured my heart out, I felt something happen to me. The two halves of my personality were back in my head, talking to each other. The half of me that liked to get down on myself thought, *Hey, I want to be out where I can put some restraints on the other half that always wants to go off picking daisies. I want to say that you've got to complete tasks in a certain time. You've got to get up in the morning and get your work done. You cannot go off daydreaming.*

Then the other half of me said, *Yes, I need that, but I want to have some freedom to create. I don't want the other half of me to get too discouraged when things do not always have a positive conclusion.* I always knew God created everything n Heaven and earth, but the subtleties of God became clearer to me when He came to me in the night and helped me with my personality.

The parts that God temporarily placed in my subconscious came out and united with the part of me that stayed in my conscious mind. *I'm being healed by God, the first and last potter, the almighty psychiatrist, who developed my psyches,* I thought. I felt relaxed and went to sleep. For some of us, much of our immobility and resistance to renewal is seated in our psychological hang-ups.

According to Speed Leas and Paul Kittlaus, in their insightful book,

Church Fights, Managing Conflict in the Local Church, one way of identifying automatic thoughts is to provide symptom relief by teaching clients to argue with themselves, to dispute their automatic thoughts with rational thoughts in order to gain control over their feelings.[1] "Will I eat this piece of pie or won't I? (weighing the pros and cons.) The models presented in *Church Fights* can be useful so I recommend this book. I want to state man imitates God, not the other way around. God invented self-talk, not man. "Love the Lord thy God with all your heart, mind, and soul and your neighbor as thyself." That is not bad.

You may remember the television story of Cybil, a person with multiple personalities, who with a psychologist helping her to recognize and accept all parts of herself without shame, and through talk therapy with the doctor was able to unite her personalities enough to live a better life. For those of you who can remember back to the 1950's, the movie, All About Eve, Joan Woodward's character, through talk therapy which included arguing with herself, was able to except her multiple personality disorder for better results.

When I woke up, I smelled bacon cooking in the kitchen. My husband was fixing breakfast for David and letting me sleep in. I was so refreshed, I felt whole! Much of my past garbage no longer bothered me.

Since that night, reading Scripture and other Christian writings, prayer, sermons, classes, and small group meetings, have helped me learn to discern spirits. I can stay in the present and not brood about past hurts. I pray I can keep my thoughts in the present.

Now I believe I'm developing a balanced personality of Christ-like behavior, a new me. True renewal of the mind is what Paul talked about, "I was finally, truly in God, and I could feel the presence of the Spirit within me, in a defining way." The most memorable experience was when I heard the sweetest voice ever ring in my ears through the Holy Spirit: "Ah, look what Lucifer has done in my Jan's mind. How could he hurt my beautiful lamb, this creation of mine? We will make her whole."

My caregiver is my Lord. I do not need my own fleshful 'blah, blah, blah!' But I am human; I still fail and ask forgiveness. (See notes for ways to improve our communication).

ANTIDOTE AND CAREGIVER HELP

Do you communicate, or do you just talk?

Communicating is more than talking. It takes skill and can be hard for a person with a traumatic brain injury (TBI). To communicate, you need to do certain things and avoid other things.[2]

These are things you need to do:

- listen and ask questions
- take turns talking and listening
- give accurate information
- be organized and get to the point
- keep your emotions under control
- be aware of how you are affecting the other person

These are things you need to avoid:

- interrupting
- rambling
- making the other person do all of the work to keep the conversation going
- yelling
- making comments that others might think rude or mean

What happens if someone's communicating skills are not good?

- It may be "too much work" to communicate, so he or she may not try.
- Others may avoid having conversations with the person.
- It could become difficult to make or keep friends; it may be hard to find a "girlfriend" or a "boyfriend."
- It may be hard to keep a job.
- The person may not feel very good about himself or herself.
- In the end, some people start to feel isolated. This feeling can last a long time.

These are signs that a person's communication skills might need improvement:

- Conversations may be confusing to others.
- When they talk, they may give too little or too much information.
- They might sound disorganized.
- They might ramble and repeat themselves.
- They might not catch and correct errors they make when talking.
- They may get off the topic.
- They may not give enough detail.
- What they say may not be interesting.
- They may talk or process information too slowly.
- The other person may have to ask a lot of questions to keep the conversation going.
- They may not know how to use "clues" of "hints" from the other person. This includes things like gestures, eye contact, and emotions. Other hints might to how close to stand to the other person, or how loud to talk.

This chapter is a sampling from the book, *The Humpty Dumpty Syndrome,* and includes quotes from experts that could have helped out family had it been available to the brain injured and their families.[3] These sources plus the information helped as I wrote an addendum to my book *The Humpty Dumpty Syndrome* added for dissertation requirements for my doctorate with a minor in "pastoral counseling" at Florida State University.

☙ 14 ❧

Taking Care of Self

Identifying need

When and if caregivers become wise or informed enough to know they must take care of themselves to take care of others and when they attempt to do so, Satan's manipulation can be very potent. Expressions such as "what would I ever do without you" or "I couldn't make it if you weren't here" etc. are typical and often are genuinely meant; they can also be used for emotional control. It is very good to know one is appreciated but caregivers need to be educated on how and when respite is needed. Churches can help if they understand there is a problem. God is the Great Healer. We can point caregivers to Him.

Simple worship

One form of self-care is in simple worship, in merely talking to God. We can experience God's forgiveness and mercy as we examine our inner selves more clearly with a quiet mind; freely forgiving others' and ourselves as we talk to God. To care in simple worship is to provide a heart channel for God's love and understand that manifests goodness and love towards others. Then we can take the fruits from this simple worship and share it with others. We labor with joyful love working for the kingdom ever seeking the will of God. We can't build worship into spirituality. We recognize as we simply talk to God and worship Him that we are lifted up to His higher calling through grace. Joshua talks about the suffering servant. When we take on a servant role, God blesses us. (Read Joshua 2:5). He honors the "suffering servant."

The Book of Luke tells of a group of angels appeared singing, "Glory to God in the Highest, and on earth peace, good will toward men." "For unto you is born this day in the city of David a Savior, which is Christ the Lord." "Ye shall find the babe wrapped in swaddling clothes, lying in a manger." The shepherds went to Bethlehem to see the great wonder the angels announced. (Read Luke 2: 10–4)

There in a quiet manger lay the infant Jesus. Simple, quiet and peaceful as the Shepherds and animals looked in on the birthday of a King. In contrast, when the Holy Spirit was ushered into the hearts and minds of man it was anything but quiet. It was triumphant!

The "birthday" of the Christian Church was as we personally praised and worshipped Christ through the Holy Spirit rather than through a priest in the Holy of Holies. Yet, to me, somewhere between traditional structure and contemporary changes, simplicity of worship is important.

Another form of simple worship is by performing acts of mercy as we labor with joyful love in work for the Kingdom. But doing things to spread worship is only part of it. Our personhood disappears and we become lost in God. These, I believe, are the experiences we can get through simple praise and worship. This can't always be experienced when we seek the outward structured rituals of the illusion of worship. Worship is prayer. It allows us the ingredients of love and communion toward God and one another.

The most meaningful simple worship service I was ever in came unexpectedly. My health had suffered through the years of caregiving for my first husband. He passed away January 18, 1971. Often sick myself with asthma and pneumonia, I continued to he hospitalized on occasion after Bob's death. I saw an ad in the newspaper; a traditional church was offering a class on grief. However, it was on Sunday morning at the same time as my home church's worship service. I abandoned my church's safe harbor with little responsibility to try to get other help which I believed would be more satisfying to me.

Build up your faith

Amidst volumes of devouring flames, unseen yet felt, the Almighty came. No chosen non-counterfeiting servant of love can now appease this jealous God or open up a font of grace to Adam's unregenerate race. No soldier for the battlefield to tame. Without faith, the battle will remain. Faith is so simple. "Faith is not an eerie power," says Dr. Don Colbert, M.D., in his excellent book *The Bible Cure for Allergies*.[1] He says faith is not an opinion of others. Yet, some characters only have faith in their own opinions. Faith is a choice to believe God can help us overcome no matter what others think.

Our heavenly father knows that with faith we can get through the trenches in spite of destruction or harsh methods on the road to excellence. He is our Caregiver. He knows how much of the burden we can carry and God carries the rest. God walks beside us when Satan's mud is thrown at us. We can say "nuts" if Satan tells us to quit because Christ gives us power when we are saved. God gives us tools such as the Bible and the attitudes of a winner armed with his power to win spiritual battles.

Our provider is the one and only sovereign invisible God. This principle was first identified by the written visible law inspired by the invisible God (I Am, as He told Moses to tell the masses). Moses was chosen by our invisible God (I Am) to instruct the visible mankind on how to obey and do the invisible God's will.

> Through faith we understand that the worlds were framed by the Word of God, so that things which are seen were not made of things that do appear.

We can know by faith that God is sovereign, almighty in power, our ultimate caregiver and provider.

A good reference tool for ways to build up our faith is this list:

- Read the Bible more and more.
- People aren't the problem; it's the spirit behind the people.
- Minister to others with love and an open mind believing they can be healed.
- We show fruit through believing.
- Believe with our heart and it will be granted.
- Faith is not hope but we can hope and that releases faith.
- Faith is not mental belief but believing what we cannot see.
- Faith is not acceptance of a situation but in the invisible that can become visible.
- Faith is not reasoning or logic; it is hope in action.
- Faith is not a certain feeling; it's believing in what we cannot see.
- Hope is expectation of future goods.
- Faith needs hope to live.

- Hope is confidence.
- Faith is raw inspection.
- Patience is to suffer in any degree by waiting.
- Succumb under trial is not necessary. Faith believes the trial will have a good outcome,
- We won't collapse because of circumstances when we lean on God.
- Speak to the problem in the name of Jesus and it will go away.
- Patience is a quality of mind.
- Keep our mind on Christ.
- We will be obedient to God.
- Move by the Word of God.

Share your faith with others

Keeping our own faith built up by reading the Word of God daily, staying in fellowship with other believers and being mutually supportive with them, staying in attitude of prayer at all times, and taking out the Sword of Faith be bring to mind scriptures that will counteract doubt will help keep our faith strong, strong enough in fact to strengthen the faith of others. A beautiful example of that may be seen in the letter below that was written by a young girl I know named Cecelia sent to a friend facing death at a young age:

Dear Stella,

I can understand how you are feeling and I even felt that way for a split second when I was in a coma and heard the doctors tell my family there was nothing they could do for me, that I would be dead in 8 hours. I wanted to scream that I could hear them and not to give up on me but I also wanted to cry out to God asking why He wasn't taking care of me. I realized pretty quickly that He was taking care of me, just not the way I would have chosen. You see God gives us choices and sometimes we choose wrong. This saddens God because He has to suffer the consequences along with us but He loves us, so He lets us choose. He is lying right next to you in just as much pain as you are, even more actually because He has heard your cries and He has taken the pain you can't handle and left only the pain you can. If it wasn't for God, you wouldn't be here right now and I have a feeling you know that. Your last hope for survival is God, maybe He is waiting to hear you fully surrender to Him and admit that you can't do it without Him.

You have been in my prayers every night since I joined this group. I saw your post telling of all the infections starting in your liver and pancreas and it touched me because you tell of how most people suffer through liver failure. I feel awful sometimes because I went through it so quickly and didn't have the chance to question why things were happening. I find myself questioning things now but every time the questions start I look back at what God has done for me and realize that WHATEVER His plan is, it is the right one. Don't question it just give everything to Him and stop worrying.

May the angels watch over you,

Cecelia Elzerman

Liver Transplant Recipient

Within a 24-hour period, Cecelia had become sick and was about to lose her life with a failed liver. God sent a compatible liver to her and in the middle of the night, as doctors feverishly worked over her, God came aboard once again and touched the new liver so the transplant was a success.

Forgive yourself

Before he became a believer, Paul, under the law, was good at believing he was right when he was wrong in his cruelty to the Christians. He caused conflict among the Old Testament law-keepers and the Christians. Moses felt a sense of failure when he asked the Lord to relieve him of leadership in the wilderness. God's reply was that the journey to the Promised Land should continue as before. Moses ascended the sacred mountain, carrying two stone tablets that he had hewed to replace those smashed. Once again he stayed there forty days and forty nights without food or water. When he returned with the "…words of the covenant, the Ten Commandments" engraved on the tablets for the second time (the old order), Aaron and the Israelites observed that his face shone with such light that "...they were afraid to come near him." (Exodus 34:28–30, KJV)

Under the desert sun Elijah cursed the day, sat hopelessly under a tree, and asked God that he die. "I have had enough, Lord," he said. "Take my life; I am no better than my fathers." (1 Kings 19:4, KJV) Elijah felt alone in battle and powerless against the threats of Queen Jezebel. Other prophets had already been killed and he did not think there was any point in living.

God restored Elijah by changing his negative thoughts to positive ones. Rather than give up and die, Elijah was ready to serve God. He no longer considered himself along because God was with him. By changing his negative thoughts of death, Elijah served God in more powerful ways. We, too, can overcome feelings of despair, loneliness, depression, and helplessness.

Set realistic goals

On important way for caregivers to take care of ourselves is to set personal goals. That's right, personal goals—not just goals for those we are caring for. I make sure that I make a list of New Years Resolutions and then do my best to fulfill them.

Each New Year brings forth a pause in our lives-a time to reflect on unfulfilled dreams, unrealized expectations, and uncompleted tasks. As a caregiver, there are so many ups and downs, of emotions running rampant. We can find ourselves wondering why we do not have a caregiver for ourselves. What has happened to our own life? Many people use the holidays or the beginning of the New Year to gauge one's successes or failures. The new coming of each New Year ushers forth a whole new list of resolutions.

It is important for caregivers to make resolutions for themselves as well as those that they care for.

This year, make a vow to keep the following "Caregiver" resolutions:

- I will set limits.
- I will determine what I can reasonably do for my loved one and draw some boundaries for myself.
- I will accept and enlist help. Siblings, other relatives, and

neighbors often offer to lend a hand. This year, I will say "Yes" to those who offer to help and do so gratefully.

- I will not waste my energy on trying to change my loved one.
- I will learn to say "No."
- I will learn to say no to my loved one if I will be over-extending myself emotionally or physically.
- I will practice saying no in front of the mirror.
- I will accept the "Unthinkable Thoughts" as part of being human.
- It is normal to feel a sense of guilt and helplessness. When I feel this way, I am going to look at the situation from another perspective. I am going to look at what I am doing, not what I am not doing, for my loved one.
- I will find enjoyable ways to ease stress and take care of myself.
- I will find some respite care for an afternoon of self-pampering (reading a book, getting a haircut, getting my nails done, etc.).
- I will find friends to get together with at least once a week for support, chatting, diversion or even gossip.
- I will engage in regular physical activity such as visits to the gym, or a home exercise program, or an evening sports club.
- I will find something to laugh about.

—Dr. David Lowell, Catherine Sebold
National Brain Injury Association, *Caregiver Resolution* [2]

Be a soulwinner

One important way for us to regularly get outside of our own heads and look beyond our daily routines is by being a "soul winner" in our daily lives. Not only is this our Christian responsibility, but it also help us to stay aware that the overall picture is much larger than our immediate crisis.

I have found that following the guidelines listed below have helped me to keep on track.

Do's for Soul Winner

- Pray earnestly—you need the anointing of the Holy Spirit. He will convict you the one you seek to win.

- Be sincere and in earnest—these go along way to help you succeed.
- Be kind—the Spirit of Christ is an asset.
- Have some Christian literature to offer your friend.
- Be natural in manner—this places your friend more at ease. In such an atmosphere it is easier to make progress.
- Cultivate the ability to direct the conversation into spiritual channels. Let us never think it is unusual to talk about our Savior and man's need of Him.
- Seek an opportunity to do a kind deed in the name of Christ for the person you wish to win.
- Be courageous—God says, "Be not afraid," He is with you.
- Answer questions and meet excuses with God's Word.

Don'ts for Soul Winners

- Don't attract attention—Christ is the Great Attraction.
- Don't multiply texts and illusions—two or three scriptures are fine. Keep the procedure simple.
- Don't be impatient with people—you may lose a soul.
- Don't criticize any church—this will only hurt you and your cause.
- Don't hurry—it takes time to win a soul. You may have to come back again and again to win.
- Don't embarrass your friend—remember you are trying to help him/her.

Resolve conflict in healthy ways

At times, conflict with siblings or family members over how to best take care of an elderly parent or otherwise ably challenged family member will arise. Taking a look at how a conflict that Bill's sister Neva had with their mother helps illustrate how listening others and finding creative solutions helps resolve conflict. Here, Neva describes an example of the challenges facing children with elderly parents:

"Bill's mother thought her independence was being challenged, so she protested and would not cooperate. She stated that she was going to live in her own home until she died. My mother did not want me writing checks from her account to pay bills, yet she needed help," Peak recalled. "I thought she did not trust me and suspiciously thought I was trying to treat her like she was feeble minded. We hurt each other's feelings and there were many tears shed." A new program came to the rescue that is staffed by volunteers and is funded by grants and each participant's ability to pay.

The program center was open daily from 10 a.m. to 2 p.m. The paid staff consisted of a program director, a recreational director, a nurse, and two bus drivers. The center stresses medical security, social activities, transportation, good diet, hygiene, exercise, and telephone assurance. These examples of services could also be offered at a care or healing center. They helped medically through the staff nurse, who checked skin spots, blemishes, swelling, and other minor medical worries. "Socializing with the other patients is extremely comforting for my mom," says Peak. But adjustments had to be made by all parties concerned for the program to really work.

While interacting with a diversified group of individuals that crossed my path when I was writing *The Humpty Dumpty Syndrome*, I found that disputes resolved quicker if we simply stick to the issues. When we start pointing fingers at individuals or groups of people with different traditions, cultures, and styles who are not necessarily ungodly, it is threatening and can produce negativity. When I am being accused falsely, it takes much prayer, self-discipline, and emotional control for me to not begin to consider the accusers' weaknesses and point them out in return for their accusing. Although this only adds to the fire, I do not always hold my tongue. I ask for forgiveness from God and those concerned, regardless of who was at fault.

> Avoid foolish disputes… for they are unprofitable and useless.
> —Philippians 2:14, kjv

Everyone will, at some point, get into conflict. We can see it in two small children's conflict over a toy. No one taught them to pull his/her way on the toy while screaming "It's mine!" Or the child who takes password information out of mom's purse while other children look on, then participate in reading the forbidden internet information that mom's broken down code allows. Mom comes along, notices the forbidden material on the computer and asks simply "Who got in my purse." All point to the child whose hand actually got into mom's purse for the password. Of course, we get this from Adam and Eve as each passed the blame—Adam to Eve, and Eve to the serpent.

> The long-term effects on a brain injured individual or their families, or caregivers, or other support people can cause conflicts regarding treatment methods. While doing what is best for ably challenged children becomes a part of their daily lives, the burden of responsibility and care within a context of external constraints beyond parents control takes parenting beyond rational and logical bonds. It is only by trusting in God and having supernatural hope that I am able to make any sense at all out of my son's accident. Caregivers can attest to feeling this way also.[3]

When considering our approach to a possible conflict or response to impending conflict, we can keep in mind that we are all ably challenged in some way. Because the person with whom we may be headed for conflict is most certainly ably challenged in one way or the other even if the thorn in their side is not as obvious something like as ADHD, we can respond in light of the knowledge that we are called to be our brother/sister's keeper (or caregiver).

If a problem can be avoided, it should be avoided!

Jesus gives us wonderful biblical examples of how we are to respond when faced with potential conflict:

> Evil for Evil, or railing for railing: but contrariwise blessing; knowing that ye are thereunto called, that ye should inherit a blessing.
> —1 PETER 3:9, KJV

> But I say unto you, that ye resist not evil: but whosoever shall smite thee on thy right cheek, turn to him the other also.
> —MATTHEW 5:39, KJV

And through Christ's example we are also admonished:

> Who, when he was reviled, reviled not again; when he suffered, he threatened not.
> —1 PETER 2:23, KJV

Be obedient

Our acts of obedience to God, and caregiving guided by God, reflect His mercy to us, through us and into others. God cherishes obedience in our connections with Himself and overlooks the unbecoming by the grace of His son, Jesus Christ.

An example of how important it is to be obedient to the urgings from the Holy Spirit may be seen in my testimony of a time when I was struggling with faith when diagnosed with breast cancer but simple obedience God me through:

Pastor Dave speaks of "dirty diapers" in referring to Christians who seem to remain with babe-in-Christ characteristics far too long. An authentic modern-day-prophet, Dick Mills, perked me up once as he prophesized mighty things for me that fanned the flame of incredible joy in my heart. I wondered, however, what he would think if he knew my most strategic victories were over diaper rash—but a victory is a victory. I dreamed on, *God will heal me of my ADHD and Dyslexia. I'll be famous, doing profound things. I'll become a great administrator.*

But one day after tests, I was told I had breast cancer. "God," I prayed "that stuff can kill a person. I'm going the wrong way on the scale of life."

God answered, "It's okay, Jan. What you have cannot grow: it's dead. I have a purpose for your life."

I responded, "But, but God …"

Soon afterwards, the pastor gave another sermon mentioning diaper rash, citing the cure as taking our troubles to God in prayer and leaving them there.

During the message I knew that I have a tendency to leave my troubles with God for only short periods of time.

After hearing this message, I told a sister in Christ about my medical diagnosis. "Maybe there is no cancer in your breast." she suggested. "This can show when they take nodes out."

I pondered my faith.

God counseled me. "Remember Dick Mills' positive prediction for you."

Low in trust for the moment, I answered. "Who's he?"

(Shame on me—diaper rash again.)

But, obeying God, I went to a healing center and had hands laid on me by two wonderful ladies. Family, friends, and other church congregations prayed for my healing. Obedience to God overlooked much in me.

No cancer showed in the operation. Only a little pre-cancerous lymph nodes—Perfect! All in harm's way was removed. No chemo, no hair loss. Hallelujah!

My sacrifice of flesh is small in order to again give thanks and praise His holy name for His great works of steadying me. Again, thank you Lord. I'm not famous, but I am a caregiver.

Celebrate and support others' caregiving works that may be different from yours

Celebrating and supporting others' passions spreads much joy and keeps us humble. While we may tend to gravitate toward people are in circumstances to ours, broadening our horizon will keep us humble and enrich our lives. I am often surprised to learn just how passionate a person can be about something that I hadn't thought about much.

A rich example of this happened when my husband was sick and a loved family member came to visit us at a new house we had built on a strict animal control lot in the summer of 1979 and brought a dog, Albert. We were having our lawn sodded. Adding to our dog yard space dilemma, the sod was delivered while my husband was hospitalized. The lawn job could not be postponed, and the new sod would need constant watering. Sod job completed, I realized I needed extra hose and sprinkler equipment. I moved quickly to the hardware store and got what I needed. I discarded the little rubber round things not realizing they were gaskets to keep the hose from leaking. What do I know anyway? The sprinkler's water squirted out of every connection making pools of water in some spots and leaving other spots virtually dry. I tried to move the hose around, but I sunk to my knees in mud. I had not thought of purchasing sod shoes. My son's tennis rackets might do in a pinch, I reasoned, even though there was time in advance to obtain sod shoes. I did not take into consideration what my affluent neighbors in the subdivision would think.

The next day the family member brought Albert over. I would be the dog's caregiver for the afternoon. A chain fastened him to a post holding our rail fence. Nearby a hose leaked water for the sod. Off she went.

I went to the garage and tied the old tennis rackets to my feet moving the leaky hose away from the post. I attended to the business of moving other leaky hoses and sprinkler connections around the lawn.

All of a sudden, I heard a clatter in the five-bathroom neighbor's garage where they kept their garbage. Their little girl was up from her nap and wanted her tricycle. Albert made one lunge with the chain, and then a second. That did it. Out came the post from the water-softened soil. Albert took off for the garage to get into the garbage, post, chain, and all. I ran after him. One tennis racket came off, and I sank to my knee with the tennis racket flying.

"Call the dog pound!" someone shouted. "Call the police! Where is Mrs. Warrington?"

"Why is she calling me?" I crabbed, "It's only a dog." The neighbor crossed her lawn toward me with some garbage, a small child, and a dog dragging a chain and post. Stopping short of our sodden mess, she said, "Take this dog... Do you want the dog in a dog pound? I cannot hold him much longer."

"Yes, that's the answer," I yelled back, my feet stuck in the sod. "Can you wait until I get my leg out of this hole?" Albert licked my stuck legs.

In the meantime, her little girl began to pet Albert, trying to steer around the green blotches. Albert put his paws over his eyes and wagged his tail. "Don't pet that thing," the neighbor crabbed. She looked in horror! It was obviously her first close look. "What is that stuff on his skin? He hardly has any hair. Is it catching?" She was so breathless by now that her sentences tumbled out seemingly all in one.

"He's got the mange," I said "And I'm not sure of the catching part."

She glared down and dropped the chain. She grabbed her little girl's hand, scraping some garbage off her leg and left fuming. Her last words were, "Get that dog out of here!"

Fortunately, my husband came home soon after. Dog and loved one left for home, and we ended up with a beautiful lawn and against all odds, a cured dog. A wonderful dog at that. His coat of hair was soft and shiny. That was real faith. This dear loved one's caring for animals extends from when they are puppies and kittens to their animal's ancient days. I believe her animals live long because of her loving care. She and her husband take care of God's earth, also. Their flower appreciation goes from the simple to the unusual and exotic. Everything imaginable grows in their vegetable garden. They feed deer and turkey. They are genuine, not hypocritical or counterfeit nature lovers. Our caregiver Father/God washes away the dirt, pain, and illnesses of our body and soul. Then we can shine for God.

> By faith we understand that the universe was formed at God's command, so that what is seen was not made out of what was visible.
>
> —Hebrews 11:3

In the face of dangers and destruction let us praise the Lord from the heavens.

> Praise Him in the heights. Praise Him all His angels; praise Him all His hosts.
>
> —Psalm 148:1–2

I like to watch the Discovery Channel and I applaud the doctors and nurses who are doing so much with disfigurements caused from accidents or birth. One particular girl with such an unusual disease went through painful operations so she would not be stared at by others. We applaud the researchers who are helping find ways to prevent animals from transmitting diseases to humans and vice versa. To me these are porch caregivers. Indeed, we need to learn to love one another.

Stay humble

The table below describes the stark difference between people who have humbly had their self-will broken by Him so that may be more like Him and used by Him as vessel who cares for others in accordance to His will and people who are still prideful because they have not yet fallen on the Rock of the Lord Jesus so that they may be rebuilt in His image.

Humble Broken People

- Willing to yield the right to be right
- Giving spirit

- Self-denying
- Motivated to serve others
- Desire to be faithful to make others a success
- Desire to promote others
- Thrilled to be used at all, eager for others to get credit
- Rejoice when others are lifted up
- Know that they have nothing to offer God
- Humbled by how much they have to learn
- Not concerned with self at all
- Willing to risk getting close to others
- Accept personal responsibility
- Easy to be entreated
- Submission to authority
- Overwhelmed with a sense of their own spiritual need
- Compassionate, forgiving, look for the best in others
- Esteem all others as better then self
- Dependant spirit, recognize the need for others
- Surrender control, looks for the best way
- Receive criticism with a humble heart
- Concerned with being real
- All that matters is what God knows
- Dies to own reputations
- Willing to be open, transparent to others
- Willing to be exposed, nothing to lose
- Quick to admit failure and seek forgiveness
- Deal in specifics
- Grieved over the cause, root of their sins
- Takes the initiative to be reconciled
- Compare themselves with the holiness of God
- Feel desperate and in need of mercy
- Walk in the light
- Continual heart attitude of repentance
- Continually sense their need for God

PRIDEFUL UNBROKEN PEOPLE

- Focus on the failure of others
- Self-righteous, have a critical fault-finding spirit
- Look down on others

- Independent, self sufficient spirit
- Maintain control, must be my way
- ave to prove they are right
- Claim rights
- Demand support
- Self protective of time, rights, reputation
- Desire to be a success
- Desire self advancement
- Driven to be recognized, appreciated
- Wounded when others are promoted over them
- Think of what they can do for God
- Feel confident in what they know
- Self-conscious
- Quick to blame others
- Unapproachable
- Rebellious towards others authority
- Defensive when criticized
- Concerned with being "respectable"
- Concerned with what others think
- Work to maintain image, protect reputation
- Find it difficult to share spiritual needs with others
- Want to be sure nobody finds out there sins
- Have a hard time saying "I was wrong"
- Remorseful over their sin, got caught, found out
- They wait for others to come and ask
- Compare themselves to others
- Feel deserving of honor, position
- Blind to their true heart condition
- Don't think they need to repent anything
- Don't think they need revival
- The ministry is privileged to have me
- Can and will cause conflict
- When confessing sin, deal with generalities
- Keep people at arm's length

❧ 15 ❧

Identifying the Process and Legacy of Life

T HE DREADED DAY of placing David in a home arrived. It was October of 2002. This was something we thought we would never do. Another family member had checked out David's new home earlier and found it to be more than suitable. It was only ten minutes from us, but we still felt we were abandoning him. I heard a message coming from my voice through my self-talk. I walked through our house quietly.

I knew there was a message playing among the mingled voices of Bill, David, and the television. The message stood out, but not out of balance with scripture teachings. There emerged a light full of color throughout the house, then a foreboding cold on a warm day. I shut the sliding door. Grief was upon my husband and me as we waited for David's chauffer. Did we have everything? If we didn't, we could fix it by bringing other needed items to him the next day. Tears were glazing my eyes when the car pulled up. I shuddered. Beloved voices passed me over. David's brothers were there. I began weeping, as did my husband. He cast his eyes on David and his countenance fell. His tearfully expressive features were filled with sorrow. The faces of everyone spoke volumes.

We went about our tasks automatically. Where's David's suitcase? Where's his jacket? Does he have his tape player and records? We smiled through our fear for David's sake. It was getting to be late afternoon but we were all occupied with the mayhem around us. We hoped

David did not feel rejected or unwanted in this necessary move. We checked his room one last time. It looked empty now.

Bill was sobbing as we followed David to the car. Bill is an emotional man by nature. Finally, a wave goodbye sent him from our nurturing caregiver arms. Our pastor stayed all day and was supportive through the whole devastating process. We were not under-matched by each other in grief. It was agonizing. Our pastor said a prayer asking for God to help. Then I saw a light in David's old bedroom. Was this an invisible light? I hadn't turned the light-switch on.

The message within me was: "Trust in God and go unrushed toward tomorrow. It will bring good things." Then there was no light; just the light from another room making shadows around the furnishings.

My husband and I did sleep that night after telling each other how much we loved and appreciated each other.

Was I really between two worlds: The world of my husband along with David or alone with my husband after so many years?

Did I have a sense of Christian service calling me? We are retired, what can we do?

Oh, God, help me in these next days and weeks to be sensitive to our family."

More particularly, God help me hear more of your message through the Holy Spirit.

As would be expected, Bill and I did crash for a time. Bill spent a great deal of time sleeping, and I used talk therapy. I am not sure if all of the people I used, either in person or by telephone, were willing participants in my talking process. God came with His healing power though and I thank all of the individuals involved for showing concern and patience during this time of trauma. I believe a healing center, with trained Christian advisors and helpers, could have helped me overcome misplaced guilt and pain without intruding on others.

We would never have placed David elsewhere unless our backs were against the wall, we reasoned. He had to have more hands-on care than we could offer. This move allowed my husband and I to visit David and he would still be a part of our lives. Bill and I would spend the remainder of our days like most retired couples. However, when we get lonesome for David, he was near.

Infatuation may be felt quite suddenly, but love always takes time. Why? It takes time to develop and mature as the result of many experiences together. Love is built up gradually through numerous contacts and interplay of personalities. It can never be found, just growing idly by the wayside, to be plucked at will. It is the result of effort, attention, and unselfishness. It is a creation![1]

—MURRAY BANKS, *HOW TO LIVE WITH YOURSELF*

We believe David will find more caregivers and clients to love and receive love from. He loves humor and has the gift to make others laugh. As you may have noted, David has the ability to laugh at himself, and, to me, his golden nuggets spell truth. Here's a little final flavor of David:

There are three degrees of laughter. The lowest is the laughter of a man who laughs only at his own jokes. Next is the laughter of the man who laughs at the jokes of others. But the highest and finest of all is the laughter of the man who laughs at himself. For this shows the precious ability to look at oneself objectively, and if we can do that, worries have a comforting habit of diminishing in importance.[2]

A British professor has classified laughs as follows: People whose laugh has an A-A sound are cheerful and kind. An E-E sound means they are egoistic and gloomy. Children and old folks laugh I-I. O-O signifies melancholy and pessimism. And U-U is undeniably the sign of a hypocrite and cheat.[3]

"People who laugh actually live longer than those who don't laugh," declares Dr. James J. Walsh, of Fordham University. "Few persons realize that health actually varies according to the amount of laughter." If laughter could be ordered at the corner drug store, any doctor would prescribe many laughs a day.[4]

What brings tears to my eyes now is my knowing there is help for burned out caregivers. They can make a comeback. Those out of touch with God can make a comeback, also. The nurses' diagnosis that a few weeks in a quiet place to rest would soon bring my mother home to our family was the correct one, even in that year, 1941. However, the hit on mother's head seemed to have sealed my mother's doom. Since learning about blows to the head, all sorts of medication and therapy would have worked for her, had it been available then. Even though divine healing for my mother did not occur and I missed her dearly, I am still an advocate of Jesus Christ, who can give rest and restoration anywhere, can save, and can heal. Still burning in my heart is my desire to help burned-out caregivers move into and abide the peace that Jesus provides.

All my life I held close to my heart the special gifts that I mentioned earlier. My only two lovers are my two husbands; one in Heaven and the one who is at my side helping make life beautiful. I will be the bride of Christ when He comes. I continue to be attentive to simple acts of worship when I build an altar in my mind and praise and thank God, read His Word, sing a simple song, or hold his hand while I am holding the hand of another.

I believe God has helped me get to the bottom of my innermost fears. I have a choice. I can still be a caregiver perched upon a church steeple and not move forward. I can climb down from that steeple and mingle among the masses on the street and they will not notice me. I can go to church and pick up my religious habits that do not benefit Christ—or—I can except the Church and all its imperfections and do my best to help all live in Christ's name.

I sensed that, like many people, I was looking for true closure for many of life's burdens or happenings. But then I recognized that life is a process, not a series of closures. As caregivers, we want children out of diapers; we want our children to walk so we do not need to carry them—and we think that will be better; we think that when they are in school, we will have more time for ourselves; and then we think that when the children finish school, we can take a vacation. But then college tuition hits us. Oh, but our children's first job will mean they are more on their own. But, oh dear, we're going to be grandparents and our child's wedding isn't paid for yet. We try to keep our investments active for retirement; but when we finally retire, we get bored and think we need to go back to work. Then we discover our parents need assistance.

At some point, hopefully sooner than later, we learn that caregiving is a process that spans our lifetime. For some, it is fulltime care of a loved one, or maybe more than just one loved one. For others, it is caring for a pet, the environment, the community, the rights of the unborn and our freedom of religion, or the harvest field of souls—including ones' own soul.

Looking over my years, I realize that true satisfaction in this process is only possible when Jesus Christ is taking my hand. I can indeed, with faith, believe God has taken my hand. Through healing of the soul, I can fly off this perch of emotional and spiritual paralysis as I meet the challenges I will face until my life is over and I can have a Heavenly home forever.

> But they that wait upon the Lord shall renew their strength; they shall mount up with wings as eagles; they shall run, and not be weary; and they shall walk and not faint.
>
> —Isaiah 4:31

I pray: Help me God to know when to run, when to walk and when to stand still and accept your blessings.

> Be still, and know that I am God; I will be exalted among the heathen; I will be exalted in the earth.
>
> —Psalm 46:9

> Not by might nor by power, but by the spirit saith the Lord of hosts.
>
> —Zechariah 4:11

> I press toward the goal for the prize of the upward call of God in Christ Jesus.
>
> —Philippians 3:14

If you see something running like the wind trying to reach the "goal" with which to bond, don't be afraid. It is me with the Holy Spirit chasing me, trying to rescue thee. We've been on the hunt for the eternal soul of me and thee. A hunt that doesn't take a breath while trying to reach a "goal" that seems so far away. You see, Jesus is the night star that has sent me on the hunt. I'm chasing you down for, and with, Christ. If I'm a little too fast or a little too blunt, don't be afraid; for Jesus is the head of the hunt. Because I am so fast and so blunt, it may not look like I'm following Him, but I am as precious as a star to Christ:

The child in you and in me can repent. I know He can also live deep within us on this earth, which you and I were lent. Thanks be to God, I'm again a geranium in full bloom. No more lukewarmness.

Did I seem a little too fast? Was I too blunt in the hunt for the new geranium to blossom for Jesus? I've been guided by the Spirit on this hunt. ADHD chases me while I'm trying to explain Deity, God the Father, Son, and Holy Ghost. Don't be afraid. It is me looking for heaven in the sky. I chase the true Spirit as it spins in me and I try. Don't be afraid. It is the great "I Am" guiding me. Revelations 3:20: "Behold I stand at the door and knock. If anyone hears my voice and opens the door."

I have a short "to do" list to share:

- First, check to see if my four-year-old great-grandson is still on the porch (I am now a porch-watcher grandma).
- I need to write a note to my son-in-law congratulating him on getting a deer while hunting.
- My great-grandson found a Dr. Seuss book in my past treasures. I must remember to read it to him.
- I have to send a note to the new pastor believing he will do well and one to the old pastor expressing to him Godspeed.
- Let more joy in. I'm particular about which opinionative, assuming, and presuming peddlers that knock on the door of my mind I let in. The Bible doesn't say I can pound Satan into the ground with my hammer, but I can stomp on him. I'll go, go, go, go, go and tell others about Christ. I'll build my little altar and simply worship God.
- I need to take David to lunch this week.
- I must kiss my loving husband good night.
- Back on my treadmill, I did get 1600 steps in today, but tomorrow I can and will go higher.

Bill and I believe in loving your neighbor as yourself. Our door still opens and Bill stomps his feet when there is snow. We are caregivers. Come and dine to the nines with us. God kept his promise of my appointed feast. I have performed my vows; the wicked one shall pass me no more. He is utterly defeated. Behold the mountain, the feet of He who brings good tidings, He who proclaimed peace. Now we feast at the feet of Jesus, our eternal Caregiver. We do not need to settle for a cheeseburger sandwich faith when Jesus wants to bless us abundantly. One sermonizer, in describing cheeseburger religion, referred to bodies scattered in the wilderness.

Well, I certainly had my time in the wilderness but now I hear the voice of Jesus.

> I will come into Him and dine with Him and He with me.
> —REVELATIONS 3:20

You are welcome in Jesus, and that ain't "MAYBE"!

Notes

INTRODUCTION

1. Janette Warrington, *The Humpty Dumpty Syndrome* (Houston, Tx.: HDI Publishers, 1997).

CHAPTER 3
RENEWING LIFE IN CHRIST

1. Watchman Nee, *The Spirit-Filled Man* (Anaheim, Ca.: Living Stream Publishers, 1992), 635.

CHAPTER 4
UNMASKING THE WOUNDS OF THE PAST

1. Muriel James and Dorothy Jongeward, *Born to Win* (New York: Addison-Wesley Publishing House, 1996).

CHAPTER 10
PICKING UP THE PIECES

1. Conrad W. Baars, MD, *Feeling and Healing Your Emotions* (Gainsville, Fl.: Bridge-Logos Publishers, 1997)
2. David deBronkart, *The Edison Trait* (South Paris, Me.: Park Street Press, 2003).

CHAPTER 11
GROWING UP IN CHRIST

1. Dave Williams, *Growing Up in God's Family* (Lansing, Michigan: Decapolis Publishing, 1998), 21.
2. Dave Williams, *The New Life...The Start of Something Wonderful!* (Lansing, Michigan: Decapolis Publishing, 1986).

CHAPTER 12
RECEIVING HELP IN THE CHURCH

1. Dr. Harold Shindoll, *Grace and Sovereignty of God* (Lake Hurst, FL: Wing of Truth Productions, 1989).
2. Brad Watson, *Is it Lust or Legalism?* (Orlando, Fl.: Xulon Press, 2002).
3. Larry Crabb, *Connecting*, (Nashville, Tenn.: Thomas Nelson, 1997).
4. Ross G. Menzies and Padmal deSilva, *Obsessive Compulsive Disorder: Theory, Research, and Treatment* (John Wiley & Sons, 2002).

CHAPTER 13
LEARNING TO HEAR THE VOICE OF GOD
IN SELF-TALK

1. Speed Leas and Paul Kittlaus, *Church Fights: Managing Conflict in the Local Church* (Louisville, Ky.: Westminster John Knox Press, 1973)
2. Used with permission from *Thinking Ahead—A Rocky Mountain Regional Brain Injury System Publication* (www.craighospital.org)
3. Janette Warrington, *The Humpty Dumpty Syndrome*.

CHAPTER 14
TAKING CARE OF SELF

1. Don Colbert, MD, *The Bible Cure for Allergies* (Lake Mary, Fl.: Siloam Publishing).
2. David Lowell and Catherine Sebold, *Caregiver Resolution* (National Brain Injury Association).
3. Rosemarie S. Cook, *Counseling Families of Children With Disabilities*, vol. 25, *Resources for Christian Counseling* (Nashville, Tenn.: Word, Inc., 1983).

CHAPTER 15
IDENTIFYING THE PROCESS AND LEGACY OF LIFE

1. Murray Banks, *How to Live with Yourself* (New York: Prentice-Hall, 1951).
2. *Christian Leader's Golden Treasury* (New York: Grosset and Dunlap, 1955).
3. Ibid.
4. Ibid.

09/12/2022 4:12AM September 12, 2022
(Day after MCOC Church Retreat)

Books to note:
"A caregivers triumph" by: Janette Warrington.
"Discerning The Voice of God" by: Priscilla Schirer
"Call to Discernment" by: Dean Bradley
The
"Man's Search For Meaning" by: Viktor E. Frankl

** (this one came up 2x in thast few days) **

Side Note:
9-11-2022
Of all days, MY husband turns on
a Priscilla Shrier interview on TBN
Youtube (& w/out knowing) this
interview she is discussing her

"Discerning The Voice of God"
Book & study.

(which I did with my intentional womens
bookclub
!W
This was not a mistake!!!)
AMEN! Thank You Jesu

9-12-2022 4:44 AM